The Thing We Call 'I'

VERE MENZIE

CONTENTS

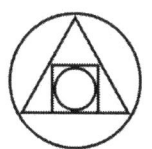

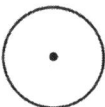

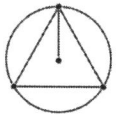

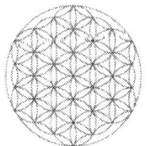

PREFACE

From your earliest memory you will be aware of that nostalgic feeling of being young, carefree and in awe of all that is. Nostalgia is a peculiarly emotional sensation, as you tend to look through rose tinted glasses at how things were, even some of the negative experiences over time can tend to be cast in a much more captivating and positive light. The environment, the aromas, the barrage of sounds, these inner feelings can all be distorted as you become caught up in the moment with a melancholic sense of abandon.

This book is about observing oneself, the many life experiences, an awakening to the possibilities we might all face and the very freedom that is held by the specific choices we make in our daily lives. It may take you on a journey of self-discovery, enlighten you to known truths with a wealth of understanding to conceptualise the underlying meaning, or simply instil you with a feeling of contentment through lifting the veil of the blind, rigid, conformity that encompasses the structure of your very existence.

You may feel the outer persona is your truest nature but that couldn't be further from reality. Your very essence comes from within and is not seamlessly harboured within the mind, it is much more than that. We adorn many faces to blend perfectly into the ever changing settings we find ourselves, our thoughts, actions and even our characters are dictated by these surroundings we are placed. From the daily struggles to the most blessed of celebrations, life can show many sides to us and it is in our very interpretation of reality that the key to a harmonious existence lies. So question the topics and ponder over each shred of information, for only then will you be able to conceivably structure an honest answer to the often evasive yet much anticipated question, 'Who am I?'

You might even discover that you are much more than you believe. If you oppose certain parts, ask yourself why. Is it really you that is so against such notions or has that been formulated by the plethora of influences and belief systems you have had throughout your life? Maybe having an openness to all things and indeed life will help dispel those fixed, closed off thoughts impeding your chance to prosper. You will find it to be a considered dismantling of the false self with an awareness of how it came to be, the content could be taken as advice or simply information to carefully examine thus contemplate your own existence.

We humans become so caught up in predicting our future we neglect the present, perpetually imagining the happiness we could obtain yet we can often become lost navigating this path, eternally searching for an answer to the elusive meaning of life! Enthralled by aesthetics but blinded to the abundant beauty all around!

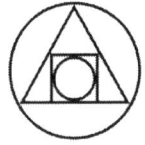

EARLY LIFE AND INHERITED BELIEFS

From the moment we are born and emerge out of this world we are merely un-sculpted blocks of marble waiting for our first indentation of the sculptor's chisel. That chisel comes in many forms but the three most prominent in the early days are the parental, societal and educational. Through these mediums our sense of morality, social understanding, dangers and beliefs are conjured, as the old adage goes 'give me the child till the age of 7 and I will show you the man'.

In these early years, through the different influences, interactions and environments we are raised in, our character as seen by others is formed. That character is our ego, our false self, this isn't who we really are or the 'I' you are told and believe you are, it is the mask we adorn and display for the outside world to see. Psychological shape shifters, we are chameleons, ever changing to suit the environment and company we keep, whether that be an overbearing parent or a free spirited teacher we tend to adjust our character introvertedly or extrovertly to these specific figures of authority and in contrast, also to a popular older friend or fellow pupil to a shy/timid younger child. The ego is eternally gripped with a desire to excel or self-preserve and will endeavour to adapt your character or output to achieve the best results possible. This narcissistic entity always has a sense of need.

- How do we look?
- How are we perceived by the world?
- How can we do things better in order to achieve more?

It is always looking for that instant gratification, a sudden release of dopamine, a short lived feel good chemical that surges through our brain activated by the reward system, which causes us to feel somewhat happy and fulfilled for a brief moment in time and as this is felt as a powerful sensation our subconscious mind will try to latch onto this feeling. It will then strive to relive this euphoria whenever the opportunity arises. We will touch on this more in the latter stages of this book.

Now from the early days that we become self-aware and start to communicate and iterate our feelings and emotions, our parents begin to teach us the rights and wrongs and how we should behave. We are bombarded with suppressions of feelings, emotions and actions.

- stop crying
- don't do that
- this isn't you
- stop getting angry

- you shouldn't have done that
- stop expressing yourself
- go to sleep
- get up
- go to the toilet
- don't eat that, eat this
- stop playing, be quiet

(Now this isn't true for every upbringing but for the most part this can be seen as the general consensus.) As instinctual as this feels to a parent raising a child we should never try to force an instinctive process or bodily function onto our child, they should be allowed to occur naturally unimpaired. Now unbeknownst to our parents they can also start to pass down inherent fears, beliefs, and behaviours that can be somewhat unwarranted. From the moment they tell us simple truths and subsequently over time learn them to be true and of course because we love and trust our next of kin then almost everything that is taught to us in our youth is then started to be taken as gospel.

Sometimes they will try to leave an impression on us of their deep rooted fears or past experiences, but their own phobias and bad experiences were a result of many factors and synchronicities personal to their own life's path and could be somewhat irrelevant to our own, but now that the subconscious mind has taken hold of those beliefs and feelings it will try at all times to prevent us from encountering such things.

Most of the time this will work to our favour, but this could also have a catastrophic and negative impact on our psyche or even the life that we live. Undoubtably our guardians will try their hardest to stop us making the same mistakes that they have previously made and will attempt to control the factors surrounding us, guide us to prosper in each endeavour and correct any discourse on the road to success they see fast approaching through similarities that had previously been shown to them on their search for success. But in doing so this can stifle and impede any chance of us finding harmony and a clear path of our own. Julius Caesar (as we are said to believe) told us 'experience is the best teacher'. This was quoted in the personal sense, yes we may ask someone else who has been in similar circumstances how their experience was, with a sense of wonderment, or if we are fretful we perhaps might ask for advice from someone close to us who, we know, has experienced the same pain and suffering and ask them how they dealt with it.

Asking for advice will always be more beneficial than having advice thrust upon you, as this type of authoritarian teachings in time loses its sense of importance and we seem to drown the sound out as white noise and the eye rolling begins. Being told an answer to a question we have not asked will always receive the same response; hence, we must have a keen interest first before advice can be accepted fully.

Now Julius Caesar may have potentially touched on a brilliant lesson! Yes experience is a great teacher as you have to live it for you to really feel it and therefore have a personal attachment to that event and because this is a personal encounter then it becomes real and you take this memory to have so much more prevalence and poignancy than a mere utterance from a friend, relative or elder. But without doubt the best lessons from life come from pain and suffering that is not to say we should become martyrs or masochists!

This simply means that when we, as we all do from time to time, experience hard times, then we should not fall into despair and depression or see these times as unlucky events and feel the universe is conspiring against us, but simply stand back for a second and ask what can I take from this, where is the lesson, how can this help me to grow?

When we are left with nothing, only then do we start to appreciate the things we already had. Only on rare occasions do we appreciate what we already do have and see the world for what it is! a truly astonishing feat that came to be through incalculable odds. We are reminded of just what we have through charitable organisations or seeing someone go through a traumatic and harrowing experience. It is in these brief instances that we say to ourselves, "yes we are lucky!" We have so much more than the person next to us, this can sometimes be a strong enough mental shake that we feel compelled to help our fellow beings as opposed to looking at someone who has much more than us and striving to achieve what they have.

'Good character is not formed in a week or month it is created little by little day by day protracted and patient effort is needed to develop good character.' Heraclitus.

We are taught from the moment we are born to stand alone and be counted, for then we must surely be individuals with a character of our own. We are given a name - this way we can be singled out. Then we are pigeon holed, whether that be for having bright red hair or golden luscious locks, by how tall or short we might possibly turn out to be, for the intelligence we show, how early we started to walk and talk, from when we became potty trained or from the first time we were able to write our own name. We then begin to construct this false sense of 'I' and start to believe in this fabricated self, painting a picture in our own minds of what we are and over time firmly becoming that concocted personality. It could be an outgoing audacious person or an introvertly inconspicuous one. We could perhaps be a predominantly upbeat, humorous type of character with a lust for life. Or a down, quiet, sensible type, the latter taking place because of the experiences and life that person lead and the influences that surrounded them. This could be down to an overbearing strict parent, or not mixing with similar aged children growing up and so not learning the social skills needed to fully function in society in contrast to the confident child who may have had a freer rein when it came to discipline, had many siblings, cousins, family members or friends from an early age and adapted well to social structures – all this is obviously a huge benefit when entering into adulthood.

Just to touch momentarily on an important subject of recent times, there has been much debate over the last few decades - possibly the last few centuries! - in regards to such topics as sexual orientation and gender identification. This could be down to many factors, but the most reasonable one to consider is that it is the result of an instinctual/biological crossover in the early development of the foetus's brain structure. All human individuals – whether they have an XX, an XY, or an atypical sex chromosome combination – begin their development from the same starting point. During early development, the gonads of the foetus remain undifferentiated; that is, all foetal genitalia are the same and are phenotypically female. After approximately 6 to 7 weeks of gestation, however, the expression of a gene on the Y chromosome induces changes that then result in the development of the testes. Thus, this gene is singularly important in inducing testis development. The production of testosterone at about 9 weeks of gestation results in the development of the reproductive tract and the masculinization (the normal development of the male sex characteristics) of the brain and genitalia.

In contrast to the role of the foetal testis in differentiation of a male genital tract and external genitalia in utero, foetal ovarian secretions are not required for female sex differentiation. As these details point out, the basic differences between the sexes begin in the womb. This might seem all very scientific and is in no way inclusive throughout the narrative of the book, but is worth contemplating nonetheless! Because of the many factors such as our genetic make-up, inherited traits, sexual attraction and hormonal over/under production during pubescence, regardless of our bodily presence our mind's identification could become somewhat polar opposite to this! It isn't as farfetched as some believe. It is instinctual, we are neither male nor female spiritually it is only our reality that makes it so, this is not to agree or disagree with any particular premise as the relevance of this matters not! The distinctiveness/individualism is what should be celebrated, isn't that the point to life? The unique and defining qualities!

Identical twins

Although we may have very similar upbringings to someone else we could become total opposites when it comes to our character. Take identical twins, for instance. Even though they are indistinguishable from a physical/biological aspect it may take only a few brief moments of conversation to be able to tell them apart. Subtle differences; height, speech, interests, who was the first born, the older child. Even though only minutes might separate them in age, the first born will always be viewed by the surrounding family and indeed society as the leader, the responsible twin in a fashion, whether overtly true or not. From their individual tastes to their manner, all are differing factors.

This shows how the people and influences around each of us shape and create a character and so the persona we come to believe we are.

Three siblings

Let's take three brothers or sisters, for instance, we find more often that the older child is the responsible one, the middle child or as it has been coined the 'forgotten/invisible' child and the youngest being the baby of the family.

The older/first born child inevitably goes through life's big events first, first day at school, first to graduate, first to get into a relationship, first to pass their driving test and first to find a career (not in every case but for the purpose of this analogy let's go with this general feeling).

Now the parents see each event as special and new so look at their first born with admiration and sympathy for having to lead the path for the rest of the siblings, but like a double edged sword they also look upon the older child with regret and remorse for the mistakes that they may have made due to being a first-time parent and a novice at raising children, wishing they could have performed certain aspects differently.

Let us now come to the second/middle child. This child is a chance for the parents to remedy the faults they made with their first, and so righting any wrongs. As the old saying goes 'practice makes perfect'. This child will go through the same events as their older sibling but because the mother and father have seen it all before, the mystique and attention is somewhat lost and because they avidly tried to rectify the mistakes they previously made, the regret and remorse isn't felt the same as they feel this child has unknowingly had an advantage over the older child and is subsequently left to their own devices, as the worry of them staying out with friends, for example, when old enough to do so isn't as scary a thought and does not register with the same importance as before, hence the 'forgotten' part of the phrase.

Then we get to the last born, the baby of the family who, from the day they were born throughout their life will always be looked upon as the baby and given slight advantageous attention as a result. They will be shown much more empathy and sympathy due to this, having two older brothers or sisters who have led the way and can be looked upon for advice, help and even protection can be a huge benefit.

The downfall to this is that the parents and other members of the family around them will not show the same respect and allow them to fend for their own in the same way they did with the previous children. They can become mollycoddled or wrapped in cotton wool to use a better turn of phrase. This can impede their independence, thus hamper their own life's path. The variations can be vast but for the benefit of a consensus on the things to be, it would be much more prevalent to give just a few scenarios.

An only child

Often categorised as the 'spoilt child', we can start to look at the word association here as we will do with many other words and phrases throughout the chapters. We hear 'spoilt child' and conjure images of an impetuous, needy brat with greedy morals and an early onset of egotistical behaviour. This can be and is unfairly due, as we have discussed previously. In a sense, this child was manufactured more so with the best intentions at heart.

To spoil something is to ruin it - as when we spoil food and allow it to go out of date we let that happen and no longer desire it – society, essentially, performs the same act here to the child, through no knowing fault of their next of kin, they, through many factors, contribute to the make-up of this child's personality and with interactions with extended family, friends and the public at large this only serves to solidify the character we have of said child. Take, for example, a young child who doesn't appear to be self-aware when seen playing, dancing or even singing. We can begin to cherish those moments and warm to the way they were unaware of what they were doing whilst performing with such sheer self-abandonment, but as soon as we are conscious that the child is self-aware and has an audience we soon see this as ingenuine, on that account we think the child is showing off which can be used in many interactions we have throughout our lives.

Going back to the only child, we can label them too severely from an early age and see them in exactly the same light as the larger than life show-off child mentioned previously. This is an assumption in most cases, we never stop to think why the youngster is behaving in certain ways.

Let's go through some of the reasons behind this melting pot of the child's character – firstly they fall into two categories:

1. they are the first born referring back to the point of the first child being the responsible one who has to be the first one in that newly formed family to go through life's major events

2. they are also the baby of the family - looked upon with wide eyes, they get the extra attention, and because they are the only child any unintentional mistakes the new parents make towards the upbringing cannot be rectified with a second child therefore some of the guilt and regrets remain, so a lot of sympathy stays with their child through the years.

Over-compensation accounts for a lot of the traits we see with a spoilt child too, never saying no, always buying the things they want and over protection. Needless to say, there is no competition with rival siblings for attention and so the purse strings are not as stretched as a family's would be with more brothers and sisters.

Nonetheless, the family do what they think is right but the morality is often lacking within this child's consciousness as they have not been exposed to certain moral highlighting events and truths that a family of brothers and sisters will encounter, the main one being sharing and the importance/benefit this can give to a person later in life's social structure.

We can now look at some of the more surprising positive traits of an only child. The ability to be self-sufficient (self-play) which can lead to an independent personality. We find them to be much more confident in adulthood, have leadership skills, a higher sense of privacy and lastly utter perfectionists. The most peculiar thing is the universe has an uncanny way of balancing things out. The trick is to home in on the upsides and further develop these positive traits.

Single parent-child/children

The last scenario we will look at is the single parent-child/children relationship and some of the profound effects this can have on children and the adults they become through the character and psyche that is formed in these early years. This is not to say that being a single parent is in any way, shape or form detrimental to a child's psyche and should not lead to any long-lasting negative effects! If anything the child will build strength of character from a single parent in most cases. First we could have a parent who prematurely dies, this harrowing experience will have numerous effects on a child and a longing through their life, an obvious missing part whether that be in love, protection or guidance. They will see other children's mums and dads interact with them, it could be as simple as either of them taking them to a sports game, watching them play, giving them a cuddle, this will remind the child of just what they have missed out on as a result of losing their parent. A hard fact of life always and the child can grow to question why them, why did the universe conspire to take their parent! What had they done to deserve this? In time and with maturity they begin to come to terms with this raw emotion and learn to accept it, albeit with a small sense of emptiness within them.

As hard as it is to lose a parent at any age, to lose a parent at such a young age is heart-breaking and there are certain aspects that will need to be compensated. In time the transformation and maturity of the child turning from a juvenile into an adolescent will open their eyes to the realisation that it was out of their hands thus learn to accept the tragedy. When it comes to a family split on the other hand it is all in the detail – the manner of a break-up, did the child witness any of the negative talk, rows or name calling? Was it an amicable break-up? Was it a result of an affair? Many differing playouts can be seen within a family break-up. Let us look at these in more detail and some of the negative impacts that can affect a youngster's mind as a result.

A break-up due to an affair

The child's mind will immediately try to understand the reasons why mum and dad have split up. They will feel lesser as a result due to them feeling emotions of inadequacy for themselves and even the parent left behind, they could have tendencies to rebel against the parent who left or, much more evident to the parent left behind, they might even see this parent figure as hopeless, somewhat tainted for their father or mother leaving them. They will feel guilt and sympathy towards this parent and might even come to the conclusion that they were the cause of the inevitable break-up!

Self-blame is common when we do not understand the meaning as to why things happen. This child will hold these feelings deep within their subconscious and might become closed off as a result, therefore detaching themselves from the people around them. In some case's the child might actually be internally blamed by the parent left to pick up the pieces. The parent could well harbour feelings of disdain for them, maybe because they see their ex-partner who has left in the child's eyes which can cause many mixed emotions. They love the child and will consciously know their baby is going through the same hurt and pain, but as we have already mentioned the subconscious mind is the aggressor and powerhouse in the brain and with it being the emotional brain it is very hard for us to override it. Consequently a parent might lash out at the child/children because of this.

Guilt and shame will come to the forefront of this parent and they will try to right the wrongs from this but it will be a never-ending battle for the first few months maybe years until time heals the raw wounds from the split. Most of the time the parent who left still wants contact with the child/children they ultimately had to leave behind, but are aware of just what a tricky process is in store for them as the loving partner they left will be hurt, could show signs of hatred and, to poke the metaphoric bear in this situation, will only serve to antagonise and then run the risk of retribution coming from the scorned, heartbroken parent/ex-partner. Revenge is classic in these cases, because the pride of the loved one picking up the pieces may have taken such a beating they feel the need to emerge from this showing dominance and power and so wish to give a swift kick (metaphorically!) to the deceitful ex in the process. It wouldn't/couldn't hurt could it? They know the first and biggest thing that will hurt them is access to their child/children therefore they perform a pincer move. Revenge for the way they left as a counter-attack and power over their ex-partner to help with the healing process of their damaged pride. Another hang up from the ego.

The lasting damage that can come with a less than amicable break-up, can stay in the deepest depths of a child's mind, causing powerfully negative behavioural changes, impeding their development and chances of a clean start, social issues, relationship issues, even everyday functionality can be hindered by this event.

We have to be present with our thoughts for only then can we justify our actions, to have a child with someone and maybe within a year find we no longer feel the same and move on only leaves a sense of neglect. Of course, we cannot get it right every time and, in this instance, we ought to come to a civil agreement with sincerity being the core ingredient. Okay, but what about the partner who did not want to change or who has been left behind?

As upsetting as it may seem at the time with our passions governing our thoughts, ultimately this communion would serve that person no meaningful purpose in the next chapter and so being mindful that these events are out of our control. The mastery of one's own psyche will assist in showing that person why this unfortunate pivotal bump in the road came to be. Only by understanding and reasoning with this set of circumstances can we hope to protect the beautiful people from the negative effects and consequences that a separation may have. This will also go some way in helping a person let go of their ego. This is not to discredit the many lasting relationships still enjoyed by happy couples all around, but to purely focus on the dynamics of break-ups as that is where the persistent issues lie.

In the meantime when it comes to inevitable break-ups, on occasions it would be more beneficial to ourselves and those around us to not take things too personal, allow events to unfold and see why they had to happen for us to grow and move on to better times. This may never apply to you but it is a point that should be addressed nonetheless as we have all bore witness to such things whether it be our close friends or family, maybe it has even affected you as a child too. Sometimes people who come from fractious families can either take a longer time to find stability in their life or can gain independence from an earlier age as a result, so long as the impact is lessened considerably.

Parental and family ties, do they hold us back? Are we guilted into doing things we would much rather not? We should never feel guilty for anything we do! What we do is the outcome of many factors and we are unaware of exactly why, we often take time to plan a strategy of how to go about things, scenarios of how the future might play out. But when it comes to pass, most of the time we act spontaneously.

Do our parents force us into things, religion, sports, education, professions? If so why? Is it because they think that is the right thing to do? Are we thought to be too immature to really know what we want? Is it because they want the best for us? As we have already talked about, if they went through the same thing with their parents, do they subconsciously identify with this notion? Maybe a break in the cycle from a subjective manner is what we should teach our early generations.

We can also inherit prejudices from our elders that could have possibly been passed down to them or have risen from their own bad experiences, always be mindful of this fact!

Education

Within our schooling we are sometimes made to learn certain subjects that are of no personal interest and hold little to no relevance to ourselves, we can then be forcibly chastised for submitting poor quality work as our inspiration can be lacking. We are all unique in the sense that the universe wishes to observe itself through many different spectrums therefore, we must all offer some creative individuality and so to learn mundane topics through personal preferences will undoubtedly cause frustration and result in poor study time, this could be seen as a caveat to the future of education.

Schooling subtly teaches children about conformity and social structure. They ultimately want the child to grow into civilised adults that have something to offer society but not necessarily humanity. Schoolchildren are told to stop daydreaming whilst staring out of the window, essentially what the teacher is saying is stop thinking! Stop being yourself! Conform to our ways of thinking and our understandings and concepts. We have to believe that we all have a part to play. Whether brain structurally someone is different to someone else or thought to be lacking intelligence, - that maybe so, academically! - but that person might just have a different calling in life which may be far removed from the likes of calculus, biology or even literature.

Schooling can be beautiful if the teacher's goal is genuine. The educational system is essentially a governing body and you have to assume that the goal is to produce submissive conformists with a wealth of knowledge that will enhance society through monetary structures. Also, advances in science and exploitive endeavours which have positive and negative aspects always attract empathy as that is felt to be correct and righteous as opposed to a chaotic senseless society in disarray that is falling by the wayside due to unrest and a fractious banking system.

We have to harness each individual's strengths and help them to flourish instead of stifling the very thing that might interest them and turn out to be their faculty, a teacher can quickly lose their student's attention as their thoughts precariously wander into the abyss of time as the captivating elements that should have been present during lesson time fall far short of the intended mark.

It can be a shame for the tutor as they have to stick to a strict syllabus laid out before them, they can incorporate as much fun as they wish but if the child is not gripped by the subject matter they will only show a feigned interest. So to punish a child that does not have a keen interest or isn't au fait with a certain subject the populous deem worthy and of great significance will only result in feelings of inadequacy followed by an overly critical sense of self and many restless nights. A brief account of subjects that will help guide us through life should suffice.

Once we alter the perceptions through a change in the context of a subject, we also change the rigidity of a fixed mindset. We often hear how the real life lessons, the basics, should be taught, like how to obtain a mortgage, file a tax return or ways to increase your credit score, but are rarely integrated into the curriculum. Possibly allowing the child to choose from a wider range of subjects that best suit their individual strengths will have the most meaningful results and so serve as a greater good for future generations and in turn the planet as a whole. It is imperative that we guide them in such a way to be ready and able to pull them back from the cliff edge but not stifle them enough to stop them embarking and ascending the great mountain because of the perils ahead. For only then can we help to reform the future of humanity's collective consciousness and learn to become sentient in our approach.

Religion

We can all postulate about the many differing religions, we can also find it somewhat amazing with a slight air of coincidence that if we are religious (even though small changes are made to better suit our own beliefs) most of the time we are so indoctrinated into a religious belief from an early age that those creeds stay with us for the rest of our lives and we protect said faith with all that we are, sometimes defensively, which is a subconscious human trait to do so. As we dispel any other belief system that does not tie in entirely with our own. People die for what they believe, which is somewhat heroic, it can be said! But let's now turn this on its head, to stand by a belief system with every notion and part of you is righteous, we can all agree, but it is all about the objective.

If morally you stand up for the ethical side of things - the persecuted and voiceless - then your moral compass is guiding you. If you stand for something that is taught to you without any ethical meaning, just ignorance and stubbornness, then the compass may have to be calibrated slightly.

Let's say conservatively, of the people born into religion at present, around 60% stay with that religion, 10% possibly change their religions and 30% become agnostics or atheists, this is all conjecture! But that 60% was much higher in times gone by, and to think of the countless wars and deaths that have come from this personal set of beliefs! We must objectively stand back and think what a coincidence it is then that we are born in the perfect place within a perfect religion! So to then go on and say other religions are wrong and squabble or even fight for these very arguments is incomputable and driven entirely by a person's pride, their defence mechanism will force them to action or compel them to berate a message that conflicts their own mental judgement, with opinions of condescension or that of the conveyance as pretentious drivel. We should take whatever surrounds us in a positive light like perpetual optimistic Omnists and learn to be aware of our fellow beings, as to have faith is ultimately to have hope!

To conclude this chapter, children crave undivided care and attention because of their vulnerability and instinctual nature, they are extremely under developed when they emerge due to the large cranial capacity to house their vast developing brain structure and so it would be near impossible to exit through natural labour at a less vulnerable stage in the gestation period if prolonged to a more suitable time frame.

"Children are our future" we hear this countless times and take the thought in with some understanding but never fully grasp the concept. They are the future of humanity, they are the future of this planet, it will either be held and nurtured by their very hands or could just as easily be crushed into fine particles of dust as we and our forefathers have shown. It would be wise for this importance to be taken with more significance than it presently has. They are formless pieces of clay waiting to be fashioned into beautifully natured affable adults who exude kindness and love and, most importantly, who meet conflict with reason not hostility, this is how change is made. They, we, humanity, are innocent and pure! Only external influences can cause corruption of these truths. Our upbringing has a profound effect on the lives we lead and can even dictate the paths we choose to take. Always be mindful of this very concept when the time arises for you to question your own being or how your life has turned out! You can change the course at whatever time you wish to, try to understand who you are and how you came to be, for only then will you be able to move in a different direction and begin to accept and cherish the uniqueness that is you, your personality is as unique as a fingerprint! No one else in the world has all the traits you possess, it can be akin to the variations of a deck of cards, sure there are many that share similar aspects! But simply put, there is no one is quite like you.

OUR PLACE IN THIS WORLD

In this world we have many groups of people who gravitate to a certain classification. There are introverts and extroverts and many variants in between. Introverts are said to possess such personas as shyness, a lack in confidence, humility, a soft quietness, empathy, and prefer isolation to socialising. Whilst at the other end of the spectrum we have the extroverts who are said to be confident, social, egotistical, loud, born leaders, attention seekers, which may very well be unjust! But the premise to this is, we all find our own little place in this world, a niche to call our own, somewhere to keep our likes and dispel the dislikes.

We can also make generalisations about certain groups of people – there are many races seen by this planet that offer a wealth of diversely rich cultural attributes, which should act and serve as a broadening of the mind to all others, as all are uniquely special. In these times of political correctness we tend to have a persistent worriment of being labelled and so often resist very natural utterances forever fearful that our words may be misconstrued. Racism, a prevalent subject in the modern era, is quite possibly the most absurd concoction conceived by the human species, our outer appearances and skin colours are simply genetic adaptations to the many climates and surroundings our ancestors found themselves. To single someone out for their skin colour is akin to singling somebody out for having green, blue or brown eyes.

What can seem random is actually a very ordered evolution of a species whose sole purpose it to ensure survival and to blend into the environment. It is not a race the racists oppose it is their specific practices that causes their unsettled feelings. We may too at times become ill at ease with opposing cultures and practices as they can feel alien and don't sit entirely well within our own social conducts, this is a phobia most have regarding anything foreign and strange hence the meaning behind the word xenophobia, although its description seems to add hatred into the mix when really it is all down to the fear of the unknown and is perpetuated by the subconscious. Humanity ought to start seeing what can be gained by the multitude of magnificent spectrums, as opposed to feeling what it may lose! No one comes into this world with a predisposition towards racism, they are simply born into it.

If we are fortunate enough in life, we can get to pick exactly where we would like to reside and the abode we wish to inhabit. We can also choose what career path and subsequently the job we would like to take, which we can leave at any time we wish to do so, if only it was that easy, right! The truth is as we move forward in life, we gain burdens and responsibilities which inhibit our sense of freedom and something dreamt we may like to see come to life never actually materialises. Priorities! Priorities! Priorities! The simple truth is you can do whatever you so please. Of course, that might not be an overnight type of happening but in time the small changes amount to great shifts in our existence!

The problem we all find is that we become complacent, and things start to become too familiar and settled for us to even consider a change, and with that we begin to create problems and put up certain mental barriers, the upheaval that comes with change! The grass isn't always greener! I might live to regret it! I'll feel I am letting people down! Whatever the hang up, you know deep down that we as people seem to blow the negatives way out of proportion, but appear to cast very little light on the positives. And so, however you find your situation, if a change is needed it is best practice to remind yourself that within as little as a few months, anything is indeed possible.

Society

What thoughts come to our minds when we think of the word society? Is it the social structure around us in an immediate sense? The government? The population at large or just the country we reside in?

The definition is the aggregates of people living together in a more or less ordered community. Yet we can all have our own take on this definition, the most poignant part of that description being people living together, existing together and the paradigm of this is to do so in harmony. A strange but beautiful notion as we know this to be rarely the case through eons of existence, but nevertheless it is an ideology that is pondered and longed for by the collective. The only possible way this can be achieved in its entirety is if we were all duplicates of one another as the dividing factors set before us are race, gender, religion and classes to mention but a few. Of course as we know we are all different in the biological sense from our distinctive traits and brain structures to the smallest detail or fingerprints. We're told to believe this from day dot, stand out from the crowd, set yourself apart, be careful and wary about such and such because they are different. It is rare (apart from say, in the racial and equality aspects of society) that we are told we are the same and not just meant as a powerful emotional trigger sentence created to tap into your sense of empathy and understanding but In the literal sense.

We are all the same with individual characteristic. The reason we are all the same is because we are all a collective consciousness. This statement is irrefutable. How can we not be? To touch on a later subject we are the universe observing itself from different vantage points with ever changing perspectives. This can sound preachy and a bit naive at the same time to a robust society with a strong dogma - but for the purpose of this discussion let's use a simple theory to try to explain why we should come to this conclusion.

Let's take the Fibonacci sequence and its derivative the golden ratio or PHI. This number 1.618 or the inverse 0.618 is used to explain many things. It can make mathematics beautiful, which sounds contradictory in every sense. The reason behind this is because when this is applied to shapes amongst other things it gives an aesthetically pleasing definitive model of said shape. This was used in ancient Greek civilizations by masterful architects to design many powerful and prominent buildings, the Parthenon atop of the Acropolis in Athens to name a classic of the time, but the amazingly clever part is that the universe uses it to, form the structure of atoms to the design of a shell or the leaves of a flower. It is everywhere - the heartbeat of nature. A simple example of this is in the financial markets. Fibonacci is used there too in a relatively powerful way to predict trend patterns in variant timescales to great effect. To utilise the ratio is to formulate 5 percentages between 0 on 100, 23.6% 38.2% 50% 61. 8% and 78.6%. Now if you are curious, try to perform a quick test, find stock on the internet of a company of your choosing and print a timescale (let's say, the last fiscal year of its price).

Now find the highest and the lowest price stock has been in that time, once you subtract the lowest price from the highest price you will be left with a figure. Using the percentages previously stated, find the numeric value for each percentage of this figure. You will now be left with five separate figures at this point. Add back the lowest price to each of these and on the printed chart mark these five numbers on the side. Now draw horizontal lines across. Here is where it starts to get a little strange but interesting. What you will now find is how the price through the year tends to gravitate towards these lines, hover around or move up and down to the other tiers.

Given that thousands if not millions of transactions have taken place over this amount of time we can conclude that we as a whole are one consciousness and intertwined with this golden ratio. There are many other forms and happenings to show this web of consciousness that will be made clear later on, trends, fashion are all simple ways to see humanity is a whole. You might think this is simply following the crowd and an easy way to form popularity on an individual level, but it is all thinking and being together!

The ego works hard at this with regards to fashion and trends, these things were started off by a creative person to stand out, to be different. Regrettably, this takes a colossal motion from the population and a mass trend ensues which is a peculiar paradox as the words we conjure up of someone or something that is different a lot of the time is strange, weird, odd. Sometimes when we don't understand someone or something we will forcibly cause them/it to be outcast, the double edged sword is hypocritically that we glorify certain individuals for standing out from the crowd for being an individual and in certain cases we may even begin to idolise them.

The complexities of who we are, based on the many faces we show whilst entering into alternate social settings can cause behaviours we hadn't anticipated on, a need to be accepted even liked by our social group can cause us to develop different characteristic traits. The biggest dictator of this being peer pressure. This can help us perform great feats when trying to push ourselves to feel part of a clan, a band of brothers or sisterhood, a revolution that opposes the establishments oppressions. Although it can also have an overwhelmingly negative response to directly linked to our own feelings of acceptance and can serve in forcing a person to perform certain actions that go against every moral fibre in their body. This is the reason many people start smoking or take their first drink of alcohol or resort to vandalism and bullying. They all stem from the fear of becoming outcast in our adolescence. This migrates to adulthood through how we are perceived by others. It may be the parents in the school yard or trying to keep up with the Joneses and so buying our children the latest designer gear thus saving the child from any ridicule and persecution or even embarrassment for you as the parent! Getting the newest model of car or phone, adding value to our houses to display our wealth and success to the neighbours, going against our values in the workplace to gain favour with management and maybe take an opportunity to climb the career ladder and with it the ever prominent social ladder too! All positives, would you agree? But what can we lose in the process? Possibly ourselves!

The Hawthorne Effect

This theory states we alter our behaviour through the fact we start to become aware we are being observed by another. This can be a positive or negative response, but usually refers to a positive change, such as workers becoming more productive when observed by their boss/manager, gym-goers pushing their limits if aware of an attractive male/female watching them out of the corner of their eyes. It can also cause negative responses too, such as self-conscious episodes.

Have you ever walked down a street and upon approaching a set of traffic lights stuck on red, seen a bus full of people waiting for the green signal? The stark realisation that 'everyone on that bus is staring at me!' can cause a funny sensation. It can make our hearts race, we start to think of the attire we are adorning, is our hair a mess, do we look okay, then the rigid, wooden walking gait starts to be developed through the paranoid tension we impose on ourselves. The humorous aspect to it being, when we do gain the courage to take that sneaky glance at the bus window everyone on there is too preoccupied on their phones or in deep conversation to even notice you. Someone may glance back at you too but only in a mindless manner, not particularly focused directly upon you and in no orderly observing fashion! It could be you it could be an inanimate object or they are too busy being self-conscious themselves to even notice your presence.

Another situation this seems to happen is when we have a crush on someone either in school, at work or even on our commute to work, as soon as we catch them staring at us we start to bumble our way around, lose the conversation we are having and become all round nervous wrecks. You might say we try too hard to impress.

This ability to sense when we are being observed without fully witnessing is often referred to as our sixth sense and there may be something behind that namely intuition in a mystical sense, but the most probable cause is our subconscious mind. Even though we are consciously in conversation with somebody or deeply immersed in a book just because our mindful focus is captivated by the task in hand our instinctual/emotional mind is always wary of a threat and so acts as our lookout forever scrutinising the surroundings, persistently watching for any pending danger fast approaching, none dissimilar to an antelope on high alert whilst quenching its thirst at a watering hole.

People are driven by acceptance, many are driven by popularity and in a constant loop of attention seeking and that's okay as there is always a reason behind this, insecurity being the most likely culprit. Therefore it would not be wise or fair to show disdain for these members of our social group but instead show reason, show understanding, for this is the only way to help them help themselves. This will allow them to take off this mask that has been inhibiting the world from seeing who that individual really is. Nurture their emotions, assist in helping them out of this soft false shell they have found themselves in. When we are not shown much attention in our youth and finally realise later on in life we can obtain it for ourselves it can become a child in a candy store type of story.

A substantial amount of people in this day and age seem to have no awareness of who they are, and of the impact their actions can have upon others or if they do they treat the other person with contempt, as a hindrance or a nuisance, forever getting in the way of their life. We should see fellow beings as extensions of ourselves. They are no less nor more important than ourselves. The old saying 'treat others as you would like to be treated' seems to have lost some of its strong connotations of late, a universal connection has to exist!

Take disabilities or disfigurements for example. Although a huge shift has occurred in acceptance and empathy over the last few decades, our approach to the less fortunate can still seem patronised at times, people with disabilities don't want to be categorised or showered with sympathy they want to be viewed as equal. We think of a person who has a disability as unfortunate, less equal, the unfairness of it all, we can fall into the trap of trying to look charitable and the likability of showing the great deeds we do in order for us to gain emotional advantage over others. It is true that certain aspects of a disability is less advantageous and it can instil sorrow or guilt in the able bodied, but we do not have wings and so we cannot fly like the majestic condor, we do not have gills and cannot dive to the deepest depths of the ocean on one breath without the assistance of a submersible. It is in the uniqueness of others that there lies the beauty. A balance over time will occur, we are in an eternal search for power over this balance and need not have this struggle of the mind.

We have been conditioned to applaud beauty from aesthetics and display shame through so called ugliness as a result of the ego. Those who have not been blessed with this shallow façade of a gift may have a vantage point that vastly outshines all others as a result. Don't just love people for being them, love them for being you! For they are the people that hold beauty without prejudice, their blessings might not be skin deep but they do shine right through to their core. We can all, with wealth, change the outer appearance, but for what? Some will say confidence! Okay, but if this is where you are searching for answers then you may have become blind to the truth, and so that search will be rendered futile. Once the fake exterior has been taken off, that person is still that person, but isn't getting the applause from their malevolent friend or isn't winning any popularity contest. Nothing in this world ought to be viewed as a competition! Yes if you feel you will gain something from pushing yourself then that's okay, but trying to gain advantage over others through beauty when your morality and spirit is lacking direction is like willing your left leg to move faster than your right. And so would make no sense.

Periods of solitary

Many of us cannot seem to allow ourselves to be alone with our own thoughts. We all have to have a constant stimuli to block the thinking mind out - this is called mindlessness, something we can all hold our hands up to. But if we are eternally in this state we will not enhance any particular part of our life.

A constant barrage of visual and audible images and sounds to save ourselves from our own self and the now can only halt our mental peace and freedom of will. If boredom and loneliness is instilled in you when you have time on your own hands then you are very much keeping the wrong company and your own interests can suffer as a result. Imagine being the only person in your social group you choose not to spend any time with! It is certainly food for thought.

If time is a precious commodity then surely life is to be lived and if we waste a sizeable part of that time trying to occupy our racing minds then that part of our lives will become artificial and could just as well be spent in a visual futuristic flotation tank. Technological addiction! To many it is a frightening thought to think about losing their technological devices, some will even place dares as to how long they could abstain from their smartphone, television and computer? A week or two for a certain amount of money!

Everything in its own little way should be enjoyable. But we should seek out nature and adventure as much as possible. It would be a pointless utterance to ever say we are bored, when a short walk to the nearest window can show us all the wonderous elements of life outside the confines of our dwellings.

Technology has helped us efficiently save tireless

amounts of time from our daily lives and yet we choose to spend that time in a state of persistent boredom, so we play video games, watch films or go on social media. We may stay connected via the ethernet connection, but at the same time we are losing our connection with the ether, the internet has opened up the world to us all, yet we choose to be confined to our rooms! We conform like sitting ducks, easily manipulated by the media through cleverly precise marketing and the cycle continues!

A change might be seen in the midst, we should seek out the great outdoors and connect back with nature, yearn to observe the rolling landscape, breathe in the wilderness and savour its scent! for that is what truly helps in bringing about an inner peace.

Social classes

The social class you are born into seems to be the constant in your life. At times people can and do move up or down this hierarchy. But for the most part we tend to stay within our tier. Although the search for success keeps us on the ever spinning hamster wheel to gain status with promises of adulation along with a repertoire of temptations that if we can achieve a higher rung to this class ladder then all of our dreams could be fulfilled. The government tries its best not to allow many to rise or fall as this equilibrium has to have a certain level of balance at all times, this is how countries are run and so we come to accept this most unsettling of fact, as just a part of life.

We have some people trying to climb political or academic poles, whilst the lower classes may just be trying to obtain gainful employment, in what? Well that luxury may not have been be bestowed upon them. Security, a roof over their head, no increase to the already accrued debt, plain survival is their driving force, it is the level of the pyramid that dictates the vastness of our opportunities we can hope to receive.

The upper echelons of society are the most favoured in this game, but the plain truth is we need all walks of life to carry out all tasks! If you are a highly educated man or woman do you think the aspirations will fall upon becoming a refuse worker? Would this not seem a bit out of kilter? So, can this balance be addressed? Of course but a timely transitional process would need to occur and a fairer educational system would have to be precedent!

The truth of the matter is the falsehood that money brings us happiness! Yes to a certain point we all require a level of income to survive a comfortable life but the only sustainable way in which money can bring happiness is in the appreciation of our fortunate circumstances, helping others but never thinking we are more important no matter who we are. Whether a member of the aristocracy or stricken by poverty it matters not, it is our outlook on life and the people who are around that defines us all! Status is an imaginary ego boost, no more no less! The impetus should be on showing humility and humanity for it is a great person who can show these qualities when faced with adversity.

We can all acquire vast amounts of wealth from various backgrounds and hardships, the problem this can have is that once you are on that path sometimes it is never enough, why do so many billionaires continue to get up each morning and go to the office? You could say because of routine and a sense of purpose, the truth is status and protection! They could have the ultimate experience of life the very moment they wish to, Not to get them wrong, their hearts at times might be in the right place but only a few become true philanthropists.

To acquire many billions of dollars, pounds, euros, or yen etc and give a few tax-deductible billions away is gracious, but to truly help with honesty and a kindness of intent, without ulterior motives or ease of consciousness can be the purest thing. They may feel the need to protect their legacy or safeguard future generations but say a tenth of their wealth would be suffice for that to happen. Big banks, big pharma, big business rely on these elite figures with incredible amounts of digital cash to manipulate and profit from. Is money really the root of all evil? This is all subjective as what is good and bad in this universe is only our interpretation of the facts! A global monetary balance in time will come to fruition but only when the collective has been fully awakened, you can make the assumption they have danced with the devil but it is safe to say what is leading their motives.

Governments, how are we viewed by the powers that be? Are we just commodities? Is our purpose to provide taxes and feed the behemoth? Does there seem to be one rule for one and one rule for another, do we have condescending governmental bodies, is their role appeasement, to house establishments that serve and protect, or have they abused their role and power. In recent times it appears the left wings and right wings are both spokes of the same wheel! It is the illusion of choice; a slight of hand and subtle trick of the mind to give a falsely perccived reality.

You can tell how well a government is performing

by the level of criminality within its domain, as criminal activity is explicitly linked to the social structure it inhabits. Poverty, opportunity and social injustice all have a major role to play. When society is negligible with the vulnerable it can have a cascading effect within the fabrics of this unfortunate group of people. As a result, higher levels of crime can originate, and the domino effect continues.

Our own take on these undesirables is somewhat influenced by not only our emotions but also propaganda given out by the media as directed from the establishment, we tend to have a level of sympathy for these forgotten souls but cannot allow ourselves to forgive the acts they have committed. They become an integral part of governmental policies, this allows new laws to be passed and are the sacrificial lambs that are led to the slaughter, forever the scapegoats for the ruling classes shortcomings. It is the misdirection of funding that has the most abhorrent effect, and which inhibits their sparsely given opportunities and a chance of leading a successful wholesome existence.

Divide and conquer is a term we are all familiar with, distrust and disdain for other classes asides our own is subliminally a message to us all via governmental string pulling. This isn't a character assassination of the powers to be, but a stop check for you to leave any false beliefs and prejudices harboured within you unknowingly.

Let's say a criminal is before us and we are told about the circumstances that led to a personal conviction of said person, anger, hate, disgust, a wave of powerfully negative emotions can be set upon us and all very valid feelings upon hearing the act. So, we cast devilish guilt onto this horrendous human for being capable of such atrocities, but do we ever stop and really question just how exactly this transpired?

The furthest we go is to try to establish if they are classed as criminally insane or mentally sound. This isn't a green light to sympathise with the person after the crime! But to readdress the issues with intervention as opposed to witnessing the after-effects of the sordid events, which could have saved a lot of pain and suffering.

So let's look into how much control we all actually have and the hypocrisy of the laws, as we know law and passing sentence is derived from the defendant's intentions and so the prosecution cross examines the evidence and witnesses, and proceeds with the factual parts of the story that has to be corroborated. The prosecution then presses hard against the tangible evidence and over time a verdict is given by either a judge or ten juries after some deliberation. At this point or before depending on the verdict, the defence may opt for a plead of innocence due to the defendant showing some mental incapability, and will try to pass a plea of insanity to which a few psychologists review and interview said person, they then pass on their personal unbiased opinion. And so, if deemed mentally deficient a guilty verdict could be overturned as the emphasis of the crime cannot be directly attributed to the defendant.

Now let's take a look at another crime say a partner murders his or her husband or wife, boyfriend or girlfriend after finding out they had been unfaithful to them with another person, a peculiar (or completely regular, depending on your stance) event in the judicial system can occur. A verdict of murder can be lessened to manslaughter, and the reason? Highly emotional trauma - this is classed as a crime of passion! And so, a level of sympathy is given to the defendant, this is pivotal as the law recognises that our emotions driven by our subconscious mind can inhibit our mindful awareness and cause us to act out in an uncharacteristic manner. The only difference in this and a murder is the time frame. You see to act on instincts and emotions in the now is said to be a spontaneous reaction, and the sole guilt cannot lie at the feet of the persecuted.

Methodology also plays a vital role too, if a person carefully plans for a murder with meticulous detail, they are said to be of an evil and cunning persuasion and because of our emotional response and calculation of how intelligent this individual is, we call this premeditated murder. Let's look into the origins of this word! pre' meaning 'before', derived from the Latin word '*Prae*' and secondly, we have meditate, which has a crossover of origin. One is taken from the Latin word '*Meditari*' meaning thought out, measured, contemplated. Whilst the other is derived from '*Mederi*' meaning to heal, to cure, to remedy. Now back to the murderer!

Our feelings of empathy can be lost upon this individual because of the sheer callous way in which they planned the cruel attack, with no immediate option for pleading insanity the book can often be thrown directly at them. As a result a sense of justice prevails for the legal system and the victims' family, which is incredibly just. However, because maybe a life has been lost or abuse has taken place we are quite satisfied with our ruling of unforgivable and rightly so. But just out of curiosity let us peel back the outer layers of the perpetrator in a very candid yet meaningful way.

Could they have a slight mental disability maybe damage or disfigurements to a certain part of their brain, possibly the frontal lobe, but are still categorised as sane? Were they born into abject poverty? Were they the victim of severe bullying or abuse? Did they bear witness to abuse? Was neglect a part of their upbringing? Were they shown adequate attention whilst a pubescent? Had they been on the end of multiple rejections and setbacks? Do they have an impulsive, addictive personality? Have they been shown empathy and affection? Have they been shown trust? Did they acquire sufficient education? And finally, have they been given a chance?

This list could be endless and it may seem captious, but when it comes to blame and our convictions about the guilty, not enough importance is given to these very things as each question could be as important as the last. Society, namely the governmental approach, can be seen as two hands on after the act, but shows little effort in the intervention. If we have the dreaded bogeymen amongst us in society it can give the public something to be fearful of, it gives us a need for vital protection. Policing has the desired effect which brings up feelings of safety and security thus a peaceful sanctuary prevails. The problem arises when the government uses this very need to suggest and pass new laws and so the cycle continues, these misguided individuals have an overdue need for compassion earlier on in their life, we can directly halt the makings of a monster with more stringent and preventative steps, starting with the earliest signs with an emphasis on direct involvement and a move away from out of sight out of mind!

Giving the adequate attention the impoverished

require, and a stable and direct cash flow to the unfortunate ought to be the first port of call, we may even be able to evaluate the psychological profile of the fragile and nurture their development. This would save a lot of unnecessary pain and heartache and in time maybe social unrest and injustice will fade away into obscurity. A wishful concept it is true but an imperative one, nonetheless. We are manipulated into casting aspersions onto our fellow men/women, benefit cheats, immigrants, petty criminals and yet their very existence is a consequence of a poorly run governmental system.

Big business and big pharma, these two industries have gained a bad reputation of late, rightly or wrongly. They both have their positives and negatives, it can feel as though the state are colluding with these types of companies and to an extent they are, where taxes are concerned, but there are many other factors that have to be taken into account. We understand that big business uses extremely intelligent marketing strategies to help direct our attention to products we never knew we required. They appear to give us solutions to imaginary problems! Unless we are mindful of this they can also speak directly to our insecurities and critical self, they profess to keep us up to date with the latest technology and fashions. They try to convince us of just how much happier we may become if we just part with a small fraction of our current wealth. Speculate to accumulate isn't that the truth? This has caused over the last few decades the collapse of the small business model and the loss of countless intimate stores with their personal touch. Now ironically, we might see the possible collapse of their own superstores as a result of the growing online warehouse delivery services! The hard truth is, these big banks and big businesses are the foundation of a prosperous economy which provides an abundance of opportunities for the wider public and better times had by all, lower competitive prices which is a bonus for the consumer and larger profits for the business sector. The trap is, when we fall for the emotional response to unscrupulous advertising we have to catch ourselves, become mindfully aware of just what is it we necessarily need, not what will keep us in the trend, not what will enhance our profile, but the actual things that will serve us in our life.

Moving onto big Pharma, this sector might possibly have the worst reputation amongst any business model, why is this? These establishments' sole principle is to advance scientific cures, well that is the paradigm, the truth is profit is king in this domain. An unspoken truth about the pharmaceutical business model is thus, there are many newly fledgling pharmaceutical companies out there whom invest vast amounts of time and resources through trials and developments to get to an end goal of a potentially lifesaving cure, albeit at the many shareholders' expense. Even so, an incredible amount of heartfelt ambition goes into most medicines you purchase at the base level and in this modern world many could not live without these wonderous drugs. The problem lies within the business elements! What started off as a self-righteous moral obligation from a few scientific experts quickly turns into greed through consumerism, but as the profits are taxable kickbacks to the government, it continues to be. The relevant question you might want to ask is, how much real health education do you gain from your early education or continual studies as a layman? Apart from the odd dietary fact, sex education and a few other elements, what tangible health facts did we gain from our schooling or even after? The honest answer is that it falls remarkably short of the requirements. We all understand preventative illnesses equals smaller profits, we are given glimmers of information from scientific community at times to ease our questioning and to show sincerity but the wealth of knowledge to the average person is scarce. You could ask is that their responsibility to inform the wider public of the many ways they can assist themselves to avoid unnecessary harm through the lifestyle in which they live, but in that very question you will have formulated the answer for yourself. Just as your instincts take care of your safety most of the time, maybe the onus lies directly upon the individual to safeguard their self from needless illnesses to the best of their ability. And so the reliance on the drug companies can be of less importance (this is only in regards to the preventative aspects as once we fall perilously ill the damage has already been done!) although there are still certain steps to heal yourself after this point, providing your body with the best environments through sustenance, the correct amount of vital vitamins, minerals and essential oils. The mind's powerful healing capabilities (placebo effect) and positive living can all have an incredible healing response.

Social identity and insecurities

How do you feel you are perceived by society? What barriers can this put up and what impact can this have on your actions or social conduct? Do you feel compelled to uphold this image? Can it stop you doing what you wish? Ponder these questions for a just moment!

Now the question ought to be, do the answers even matter? Hopefully by the end of this book you will be given an insight as to why it really shouldn't! Our society's structure is built on conformity, we herald upstanding citizens and as social creatures we thrive on routine. But this can be used as a weapon against us to believe many untruths! Possibly a new law that has recently been passed is for our own good! Through media platforms, ulterior motives can be the flavour of the day. It is all rather cleverly and methodically strategised, we may lose ourselves completely if we do not find exactly who we are! For in doing this the veil will be lifted and our own intuition will take over allowing for humanity to see clearly again! Through early education we are moulded into conformists of abundant value to society. This isn't an overly negative concept, it is your awareness and understanding that can set you aside, with a level of freedom to be able to achieve anything you so wish to set your mind to.

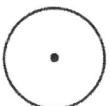

MORALITY

Morality is the rule of thumb we use to gauge an act we might participate in that does not sit entirely right with us. It is a principle concerning the distinction between right and wrong, good and bad intentions. We use the phrase 'where is your moral compass?' when we see someone close to us act in an unethical manner. At times when we venture slightly over onto the wrong side of right we can gain feelings of remorse, shame and guilt after the event, ultimately knowing the thing we did was not the right path we should have opted for. But this not so specific rule of thumb, can often be left precariously open to a wide and varied interpretation.

As we have discussed, we are taught right from wrong by the people who surround us in our youth, family, friends and teachers, but who was to say that their own take on this was correct? Or an exact science? We are coerced into action each day by our tyrant in the shadows, but it can be overthrown! Many show sincerity but this could act as a perfume masking the putrid scent of bad intentions, as we are all accustomed to the term crocodile tears. There is a fine line between something that appears as pretentious and something that is seen as evocative. It is all in the eyes of the beholder as to their take on this. It is the same with someone who seems insincere and someone who is genuine it is our prejudices towards that person that directly dictates this.

We find most of the time that it is in our teenage years that we clarify our own sense of justice and the personal association between right from wrong. A typical example is an adolescent who after being exposed to some unethical truths about veganism, vegetarianism for instance wants to then adhere to these set of principles. But they can also be persecuted by the people close to them who raised them as meat eaters and taught them that meat equals protein which would make them big and strong and also that dairy products was the best source of calcium for healthier bones and teeth. But rarely are children told the truth about the farming process or even that high protein diets can be obtained via a meat-free diet, or that milk doesn't just come from a Friesian cow that was biologically designed to yield vast quantities of milk. But that there is also a process which has to happen before that can occur.

To discuss such a matter or the previous one would negate from the sentiments of the topics we are delving into! The point being even though we are told many things at times we collectively have to ask counter questions in order for us to morally make personal decisions. The people in our inner circle even if they have our best interests at heart may still try to shield us from harrowing facts in order to protect us and our lifestyle, but not life choices! The saying may be true that 'ignorance is bliss' and to an extent this is a wonderful bit of advice when used in the correct manner, not knowing the process of the universe but trusting it explicitly is a beautiful analogy. With the same sentiment, closing our eyes and ears off to something distressing cannot be ascribed in the same way!

There is a conflict in present times with veganism, which can cause numerous fractious arguments between the carnivore and herbivore communities. You see the thing that happens is, a righteous moral individual is awakened to certain truths about meat, fur, tanning, poultry and dairy industries, to name but a few! And as they get this sudden exposure it starts to ring alarm bells in their consciousness and guilt prevails for the acts they have assisted throughout their lives up until that point. Then anger soon follows! Anger towards the industries and processes and even loved ones for allowing them blindly to be part of this appalling series of events, they now with anger, shame and guilt weighing heavy in their heart and mind, feel an overwhelming desire to right this wrong.

Their first objective is to try to make a difference and show remorse, which has to be said is a thankless task but also a commendable one! Yet because they have had a sudden realisation, they feel that the only right way to now proceed is to get all the likeminded people to have the same exposure and hopefully come to the same conclusion. But when met with a difference of opinion the opposer is treated with utter contempt and is often looked upon as ignorant and somewhat heartless and immoral for still wanting to participate in this despicable act. The truth is we all have to arrive upon this decision in our own time with relevance to ourselves if at all! We can go back to an early discussion where this is an answer those close associates never inquired about, and can be put across in a too authoritarian manner. In any regard, if we only account for our own choices and put away any guilty feelings, as this is an emotion we should never feel!

The things that come to pass happen for reasons inconceivable and so we have to just trust the process. Before the stark realisation they too were in the same spectrum, certain junctions in our lives come to us all at different intervals. If we try to cause conflict in people's lives, choices and beliefs we will ultimately come unstuck and possibly cause them to lockdown said creeds, solidifying their whole belief system.

Also, on the other side of the fence we have to show tolerance for these individuals who are making total sacrifices to adhere to this new found life choice which is an arduous journey and not to be taken lightly! But forcing opinions, trying to change other people's minds and concepts is not the true way, we have to just be aware of those around us, and allow them to find what they are looking for. Also, whenever possible and if it does not conflict with our own judgements, try to assist them. Trust in karma, trust in the universe, as what we give out, we get back in abundance isn't that the truth!

A level of sympathy has to be shown too as they might not be at that stage in their lives where they are ready for such revelations. Over ninety percent of the world's consumers of meat pay for the pleasure, as to perform the act of slaughter would be too harrowing for them, but ultimately want it doing in the most humane way possible. We all come from ancestors who were hunter gatherers, which was mostly dictated by the seasons, It was pure survival and necessity! Take vegan/vegetarian food! Or more to the point meat substitutes, which can come with a hefty price tag at times! Or purchasing fresh fruits and vegetables sometimes daily or not having sufficient knowledge in order to preserve certain foods or when you are on the lower rungs of the class ladder and just having enough food to survive is a struggle. All the factors have to be considered before any conclusion can be made, the choice aspect has to be reflected upon from a personal point of view with regards to a lot of the matters.

Firstly necessity, is it necessary? Is it genuine? Do we need that fur coat? Will I survive without my suede shoes? We have a certain level of hypocrisy when it comes to our classification of animals which we are all fully aware of. Take swatting a fly or crushing an ant for instance! These acts aren't deemed morally objectional yet when we bear witness to a horrendous act performed on a puppy or kitten shockwaves are sent out to the masses. You might have seen posters of farm animals lined up alongside cats, dogs, horses etc and a marker pen questioning where the dividing line ought to be with regards to what is seen by your eyes as food, and what is seen as a lovable pet?

We can conclude that we either associate or disassociate ourselves from the many members of the animal kingdom with relevance to consciousness. How aware is the animal? How much intelligence can it display? Does it appear to have feelings? Does it act somewhat robotic? Is it even down to the size in proportion to ourselves, as it would seem the smaller a creatures appears the less rights it has!? We are repulsed and can become incensed by the Yulin dog meat festival, yet can gleefully open up a living oyster to reveal the hidden sumptuous mother of pearl. Therefore humanity shows bias persuasions to certain individual species of animals yet not others. We have to own our acts and resolve throughout our life. Small acts, such as a meat-free meal might be all it takes to make a difference to the environment, animal welfare, the crop and water shortages in certain countries and many other beneficial factors. It is all about being present and aware of our impact upon nature.

Many countries kill animals that do not coincide with our own views. In the eastern world they hunt whales and dolphins for sustenance amongst other commodities, this to the western world can feel alien and barbaric, but it is also cultural. Pescatarians opt for a diet consisting of fish as opposed to grass fed meat, so is this a pain factor consideration? As the belief is the more intelligence an animal displays the more pain receptors they will have, right? It is widely accepted that somewhat less cognitive, intelligent animals may be slightly numb to the pain in an immediate sense as the intensity of this sensation isn't felt with the same reality as our own. To reiterate If something feels right to your own spirit, then let that guide you on how to live your life - trust intuition to be your navigator and trust not in the tormentor.

Political systems

The western world believes democracy is the fairest governmental rule we could hope for, whilst many Eastern countries opt for a communistic approach. Democracy was a gift left to us by the ancient Athenians (although it may feel as though we lost the specific blueprints many moons ago), it's premise being, that all classes of society were allowed to cast a vote and therefore all citizens' voices heard. If a member of the public was seen to have put democracy into jeopardy by the acts they had committed or even that a senator had performed unjust or was deemed to have acted in a underhanded way and so compromising his position and moral code, they by vote of the people could and indeed did use a policy not used in present times. Although the word they used is still very much relevant in today's society! That word being ostracised, this meant essentially to be outcast and forcibly sent away to foreign lands for a number of years (usually ten) to contemplate and reassess their conduct. This is the epitome of standing by your convictions and being held accountable for your actions, oh how the public face of politics would change if this policy was still in existence today.

Hypocrisy can be rife in certain aspects of our social structure, propaganda via media outlets convincing you how to act and what to believe in. So the question that springs to mind from this is, has the media's influence essentially come to make the very word 'democracy' obsolete in this era we find ourselves? The media subliminally seduces and guides you to conform to the beliefs of the state, whether you become aware of this or not. And so all opposition to their regime can be outcast by the masses as just conspiracy theorists, although there may be far-out concepts dreamt up in this circle, there will undoubtably be elements of truth and so shouldn't be shunned without careful consideration. You may work extremely hard and hand over a proportion of that cash to the state in order to help keep the country turning metaphorically. This money goes towards the education of your children, the needy and the vulnerable who are dependent on the country you reside in. Maybe healthcare too amongst other dynamic parts.

Greedy large corporations are allowed to renege on taxable profits because of a secret handshake. They seem to treat their workforce with contempt, just a number instead of an integral member with individual merit. They are allowed and revered for the environmentally destructive ways in which they obtain monetary value, pillaging natural resources that have been left to all but taken by few and the world can and has suffered irrefutably over the last few centuries, at an incredible rate as a result. The many environmentalists have been the voice of reason for the movement, chastising the global conglomerates for their unethical insincerity, an obvious commendable notion shared by a sizable amount of people on this planet. It's true the earth has been ravaged by humanity, all in the name of wealth. And it is possible it may not fully recover to what it once was, but what is apparent, is that mother nature will always reclaim what is hers if only we allot her the time in which to do so. The way to consider a change in policies is by spreading awareness, not hate or violence, but a message of moral value over the value of the currency.

Charity

Even though we have all put into a common pot to look after all walks of life within our society we are still put upon and pressured into charitable donations and time aside for helping make a difference. This is all very well and of great cause, to go against this idea could be viewed as taboo and would bring about a highly charged emotional response. But let's give it a go anyway. If the government acted according to their prior quoted values before gaining votes and stepping into office would there be a need for charity? If all the vulnerable were taken care of and there wasn't a misdirection of funding? Sure you could say that the problem has gotten out of hand, through haphazard regimes passed down for centuries to such a point that even if they implemented a stricter policy regarding charity and care for the less fortunate it would still fall quite short of what was needed. And so, we are in turn exposed to the traumatic experiences and fate many unfortunate souls have to suffer, including animals, and guilted into parting with more wealth to try to make a difference as even one life changed is worth its salt.

As moral individuals who display a benevolent side to their nature, we try to intervene and influence the path of others to feel less guilty for what we have and the fortunate circumstances we find ourselves in. Is that the only reason? Not at all, it also has a lot to do with how we are viewed, does anyone ever do anything for others without self-gain? Yes, but only a select few and only in the purest form. So, what are the many reasons we perform charitable acts? Do we do it for the kudos? Do we do it as we feel we may come into the same predicament in the future? Do we do it to impress a certain someone? Is it for a feel-good factor? Do we do it because of our empathy or understanding? Regardless of the reason the act is always commendable and only positive. But we must ask ourselves is the intent sincere? Or is it a case of one-upmanship or due to an ulterior motive? It could be something as simple as making ourselves feel better; a win-win situation. But most of the time in this generation the first thing people do is tell others of the kind acts they have been a part of. This isn't a slur on these individuals as to do so could be seen as callous, it is just an awareness check! How many times have we heard that a celebrity has donated to a charity anonymously? And yet we still find out about it! A strange concept.

Helping change the world and its inhabitants should be about the act solely, but also sharing experience and awareness not for self-gratification, it should be done entirely for the doing and not for personal gain, for this only serves one thing and the bigger that gets the harder it is to stifle in other aspects of our life. Helping others is the purest thing we can do but if we let our ego take credit, we allow the very thing that instigated the occurrence to gain momentum. If it were not for greed, selfishness and mindless endeavours would and could these injustices be a part of our social environment? Give but give freely and trust in the universe for this is the thing that will provide abundance not self-appreciation. We shouldn't feel the need for public acceptance constantly. As an ego boost or an ego trip, are both phrases we are all familiar with, charity is charity and the end result is always a beautiful one regardless of the specific aim of an individual. This is a gentle whisper to humanity.

Charity need not be viewed as a popularity platform, although we do tend to gravitate to personal causes because of the populous and uniqueness of human beings. All things in time will and should gain help from the masses, spreading positivity as well as awareness is the best practice.

Crime

What is crime and why does it exist? Crime is a person trying to obtain their desires via an immoral process/activity. These people bury the good inside them sacrificing who they are to gain status or advantage over others. The other side to this is, inequality breeds contempt and if people are not given the right to that they feel compelled to take what is not theirs, addictions stemming from the subconscious mind can play a major part too. We have discussed murder, now let's talk about the sale of narcotics!

Drug dealers rarely assess the impact of their actions, it is all about gain! Wealth and self-importance are the driving forces and power over dominion. They can be idolised even revered by the youth and can be also viewed as abhorrent characters by the older generations for the acts they commit. This culture of drug trafficking has changed most recently to that of human trafficking, sex trafficking, is this not in itself the biggest wake up call to humanity of how far out of balance the world is? The scales have been leaning unfavourably for quite some time and maybe that had to happen, if you believe all things happen for a reason then so be it, but in the same sense if that is your take on the universe then it would be wise to feel that a change is coming up in our story, for it is long overdue.

We, as people, have a concept that we are the sole influencers of our future, the truth is we have a small influence on that future but it can still be a powerful one depending on our approach and how we use the universe to walk through life and not fight the inevitable. Morality is personal, we all set our own gauges, and from time to time there can be a crossover of one individual's morals and another's, comedy for instance! This medium makes light of distressing topics to possibly make it easier to come to terms with certain unpleasant subjects. And a proportion of the audience will laugh uncontrollably, yet the remainder may become upset because it went against their moral code, we all have our own coping mechanisms and other people may simply find alternative ways of alleviating their discomfort. We should try to understand this and not take offence, they are seeing the world in a different unique light!

Intent is the main factor and we have to try to observe that as opposed to the subject matter. The more humorous aspects of life are there to be enjoyed not to be shown umbrage towards, it is a personal preference and therefore open to ridicule as it can be seen as very much subjective, but we should never be offended by it so long as it is guided by honesty. Laughter truly is the best medicine and ought to be utilised at every chance to lift a person from the dour situations they might find themselves in.

At times we can all become frustrated and possibly cause arguments or even outright conflicts because of our own beliefs and thinking our opinions matter more than someone else's. This may be for self-righteous reasons! But then self-pride takes over, fuelled by our friend the ever-persistent minion. As we all should know each and every one of us is important but no one is more important than anyone else, George Orwell's *Animal Farm* stated that we are all equal but some are more equal than others, referring to the fortunate or unfortunate classes we are born and reside in. Yes some members of society do get looked on in a more favourable light than others due to their wealth and status! But in a democratic libertarian governing system each and every voice should be heard, some people try to exist with a certain self-imposed set of rules. They try to teach themselves to become more modest and humble, to then have a conscious moral conundrum that the people they interact with may not adhere to the same beliefs by which this individual arrived upon. And so the other members of their culture may continue to go around with a sense of self-importance, not wanting to be taken for a fool or walked over, the hard working modest person quickly reverts back with the rationale and ease of conscience that this cannot possibly work in everyday life due to the fact too many people are missing the underlying message. We have to live our life by our own compass and trust in karma to help take care of the rest, not try to justify why at times we neglect the things that are important to us on a personal and spiritual level because others are opposed or ignorant to the facts, only then may we socially start to see a positive and progressive change.

Have you ever found yourself halfway through an argument then come to the realization that you may possibly be wrong but continue to fight your corner anyway? Usually this is down to shame or pride - we sometimes call this 'trying to save face'! It is refreshing when someone says, "you know what, I think you're right and maybe I am wrong". Sticking with the argument happens each and every day on a monumental scale because of self-pride and self-preservation. Call it arrogance call it ignorance, it is all about our own importance. If we just learn to take the high road and admit when we are wrong then surely the world would be a much more pleasant environment to coexist. We could also learn and grow as a result. Being wrong shouldn't be looked upon in a shameful manner not grasping what is right as a result is the wasteful element. It is the same as not asking for advice when trying something for the first time. What is the quote … 'he/she whom asks a question is a fool for a brief moment but he/she who does not remains a fool for eternity'? Wars, conflict, greed, bullying, abuse and even murder all originate from our shallow self, only when we gain a higher level of consciousness are we able to show reason and rationality in the truest form.

There are many questions we should ask ourselves!

Why do we lie? Is it a self-protecting reflex? For example, maybe we sold out and want to protect ourselves from judgement rather than it be discovered!

Why do we root for the underdog? We seem to be happy for the people who make it, because we know they have worked extra hard to acquire that life and success! And so we see them as well-rounded, humble individuals! On the other hand it may all go to their heads! At this point we begin to lose our admiration.

What about people who are given it to them on a platter (rich parents)? Why do we feel disdain, show envy and despise them? But yet hypocritically in today's times many wish for the easy road to success! Not to work hard! This might be an efficiency thought process, but also an instant gratification, high release of dopamine path, and subsequently not earnt or adaptable by that very person.

Why do we gravitate towards genuine, modest, humble souls and also the many mysterious types?

Why do we hurt others, spread hate and embody extremism?

Why do we like to witness instant karma? Is this solely a moral judgement call?

The reason for these sets of questions is for you to answer honestly to see if you can put your finger firmly on the perpetrator! We cannot view people as inherently evil, everything is circumstantial.

Is it easier to become a pleasant person when you have a comfortable life? Or can that cause internal corruption?

Is it harder when you are struggling through life and not fortunate enough to be granted the same chances as others, to keep a smile on your face and spread joy? Can this turn you into a more morally objectional person? Are there positives to be taken from this? Such as a greater sense of achievement, the many life lessons? Does this struggle help a person become more empathetic? And can it centre them or help them feel grounded?

Do you see the balance every situation presents to us? Whatever circumstances life reveals to you, remember they are only temporary, try not to get too emotionally attached to a situation because nothing in this world remains permanent.

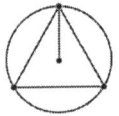

ESCAPISM

We all choose from time to time to escape from our own realities and the pressures of modern-day life. With this ever developing technological age and rapidly increasing pace of life, negative impacts are bound to spring up as a consequence. 'Every action has an equal and opposite reaction' as coined by Albert Einstein.

This generation we find ourselves, seems to be on a constant mission to try to simplify life, therefore making it more efficient. With the fallacy it will allow us to have more time on our hands to enjoy the pleasant moments and countless beautiful aspects of existence. Even though there are pro arguments for this, there is always a compromise to be made whenever trying to take a shortcut, whether that be for success or just to enrich our own reality in order to have adequate downtime to enjoy the greater things.

With the wills, desires, and pressures that come with trying to obtain our goals we can often exhaust ourselves in the process. Having a good work ethic and putting that hard work into achievements and aspirations is commendable to say the least. But the offset can somewhat compromise our enjoyment of that very success, so what we try to create are stop gaps on this road to fulfilment, to escape the monkey mind and persistent, crippling pressures we force upon ourselves.

Guilt and regret, coupled with a few setbacks, negativity and being too self-critical can form a downward trend, which can spiral out of control, so we try for brief instances on our journey to escape this anxiety filled cycle and recuperate, so that we might have the energy and strength of mind to continue in our search for the good life! There are many methods we try on this venture to balance our lives. Take a simple break away, for instance. This helps us to start living back in the present moment, be more aware and mindful of others, be more appreciative of the things we possess and reminds us of the many compromises, sacrifices we are making in order to gain security and a future for ourselves and our family.

Throughout the year when we start to feel tired on a daily basis and take on the form of zombielike daydreaming insomniac, we realise a bit of downtime could be just what the doctor ordered , so we say to our spouses or partners (or even just to ourselves) that this would be a perfect opportunity to take a much needed interval! It could be as simple as a well-planned evening out for a meal and cocktails, hiking, a weekend camping trip away from any electronic devices to reset our body clocks in nature, a cruise, a holiday abroad with its unique aromas, the terracotta roof tiles, the street life, the sandy cobble alleyways, the vast experiences and sensations encountered by its culture and the hugely beneficial effect this can have on the mind or just spending quality time with our nearest and dearest. We might take up a hobby or craft! Join a social group, plan a day in the week to talk to friends over a steaming hot cup of coffee, the list is endless but the meaning is always the same: unwind and recalibrate our internal compass so that we may press ahead with a clearer direction to head for, recalculate our options so that we do not waste vital energy on fruitless endeavours and reflect so that may become mindful of our actions! We might share our problems in this tranquil state! Mull it over and continue through with these sentiments firmly at the forefront of our minds. Learn the lesson and use it to our advantage!

We have to remember people, don't just succeed, they all follow arduous journeys in order to obtain their desired path. We so often just get to see the tip of the iceberg and that can have a negative impact on how we try to achieve our own set goals. Forcing your aspirations upon your life will have irrevocable consequences! But still we try, that's not to say people can't achieve abundance even with this uncompromising will. It is merely to say that in the process a lot of exhausting efforts and hurt can be scattered along the roadside, everything is relevant, and the frame of mind we keep from one day to the next is paramount.

When attempt after attempt starts to fail, we can begin to feel our dreams are futile and will never be achieved, a pit of depression can swiftly follow, and the realization is painfully imprinted in our subconscious! With negative talk from loved ones only solidifying this, who do so to protect you, to give you a kick up the rear and get you to come to the stark realisation that rarely do people achieve their deepest desire. They also don't want to see you hurt by the wave of setbacks and missed spent effort on pipedreams, so when all these things are compiled, we can start to feel the universe is conspiring against us and that we really don't have any backup plan, so are planted firmly in this rut, this is when the escapism can lead to irreversible repercussions, isolation and depression is an exceedingly dangerous pairing for an individual. You might turn to alcohol, drugs, gambling etc, have no real direction in your life. Then you begin to find yourself longing more and more to escape this harsh reality, and the vicious cycle continues. Without adequate help and support any one of us can find ourselves in desperate times and fall through the cracks, with masses of debt, loss of those closest to us who have gone through the perils by our side, but for self-preserving reasons they have to make a heart breaking decision, homelessness and even worse suicide can sometimes follow.

Maybe an individual had a traumatic childhood, maybe they have been psychologically disabled from birth or been in an accident that had damaged their brain structure somewhat. Whether they turn to gambling, alcohol or drugs, various other unfavourable acts can ensue from this! Stealing to feed their habits is always common, which in turn can cause them to be further cast out from society.

Prostitution is another common practice. As we are all aware with drugs we have untold dangers associated with this from criminality, gang violence, extortion to needless murder. Once again the ever present self-serving, self-appreciation entity raises its ugly head within the members of this dangerously cut throat world and the incessant need for dominance, wealth and success is forever at the helm of this crime syndicate.

The addicts, homeless or to use a collective term the undesirables in our society arrive at this juncture due to a whole manner of reasons! They require compassion, but also persistent guidance earlier in their childhood to save them from the many harrowing experiences they encounter. It is fine when we see the end product who has now slipped into criminality to forget these lost souls and turn the other cheek, but 'a stitch in time saves nine'.

When an infamous serial killer, who had previously protested his innocence, was interviewed before being put to death as he had a change of heart in his final moments of life. Possibly due to guilt, a way of repenting, or just to reach out and give the truthful account of what lead to the blood curdling crimes, ultimately knowing that it would fall predominantly on deaf ears because of the sheer disgust from the public at large. He went on to say surprisingly that he had had a wonderful upbringing with loving parents and siblings, had a great childhood with friends in his community, was somewhat popular, had no real obvious mental issues was intelligent but to an extent slightly removed from his social surroundings. He had an ideal early childhood, was seen as sound of mind, but still turned out to become a serial killer! His reason for this? Very simple, conditioning! A progressive need for more to quench his insatiable appetite.

What started off as a mild soft porn interest, quickly grew over time to a point where ever more insidious thoughts had taken full control! An overwhelming, unwavering yearning to act on these concocted ideas. At this point his conscious and subconscious minds came together to solidify this nightmarish notion! His moral compass was starting to play second fiddle. What started as a somewhat unfavourable pastime rapidly gained momentum and the boundaries soon began to be pushed ever further. This is what people do, not to say in this sense! but in other parts of their lives, we begin to get bored with our situation and start experimenting forever trying to build and harness the excitement so that we can savour it thus prevent it from dissipating.

There is always a transition that occurs for the outcasts in society from being down on their luck and looked upon with a certain amount of sympathy, to a state in which they are looked upon with any number of unfavourable inclinations! From snobbery right through to absolute hatred for the acts they have committed. Yes, there are individual schemes and charities around today which really do make a difference! But a lack of understanding from humanity's collective consciousness is more and more noticeable, as we feel today in this generation that if we tend to our own garden then morally we will be okay, a sort of, I'm all right Jack type of lifestyle, yet this just isn't sustainable.

Vices, it is true we all have a vice, isn't that what makes life interesting! Carl Jung mentioned that everybody has a shadow, a hidden self, he was of course taking about our unconscious mind, but also that there is a larger consuming dark side to ourselves than we care to believe.

We think thoughts we would much rather not at times, but this reminds us exactly what is right and what is wrong it also causes us to readjust our own sense of self. As 'Everything in moderation' is a phrase often uttered by those who partake in certain unscrupulous activities.

Chances we take

Many years ago there was a test carried out in which pigeons were placed in a box with three feeders adorning the interior wall, in the first feeder there was always an ample amount of grain. The second feeder box had a more random distribution, sometimes with grain sometimes without. The third feeder box never had any grain and so was always empty. The assumption being for survival instinct purposes a pigeon would come to favour the first box right? Wrong! The results were startling, the pigeon started to gravitate to the second random box, for the spontaneity had captured something inside the bird! This is not so dissimilar to humans, we also like to take chances in order to make our life seem just that bit more interesting, this is possibly the reason why gambling is and has been for centuries so heavily engaged in. Is it morally right to gamble? Is it right that the companies are granted permission to exploit and play on a person's habits/emotions/greed a whole range of subconscious shortcomings? It would appear so! As long as the price is right!

Back to the randomness of life, when we do not have the dark moments or bad times, or if everything was wholesome and foretold, a heaven on earth if you will, then life would get rather mundane pretty quickly. We all wish for peace, tranquillity and unity - a beautiful cohabitation - but if that were so, how many would regret that very wish? In a game of chess if either of the participants comes to the realization that within four to five moves checkmate would occur they call the game and start afresh, as to carry on would be seen as pointless and of no relevance. This is a perfect analogy for life!

When we plan too far ahead and try too hard to dictate all the aspects of our journey we start to feel the frustrations of life not performing this ultimate perfection, we need the sorrowful times as much as we need the joyful times. This gives a person that full appreciation for the things they have, it helps them to grow deep inside spiritually, this is exactly what keeps them coming back for more but as always a balance has to occur. Aldous Huxley talked about in his book, *A Brave New World* a thing called soma! A way in which we use such things to help us through the grind. In his book he says this 'there is always some delicious soma, half a gram for half-holiday, a gram for a weekend trip, 2 grams for a trip to the gorgeous East, 3 grams for a dark eternity on the moon'. This concept of soma is how Huxley described the way in which we try to escape our insufferable life. But the twist is that soma originates therefore controlled and issued by the government! A way to suppress the masses, to keep the wheels turning and alleviate pressures from the working classes.

Addictions

Addictions come in many forms but let us touch on just one of them. Smoking, this particular addiction can cause what is known as cognitive dissonance, you see we know consciously it is bad for us and is causing untold harm to our cardiovascular systems, but our subconscious mind overpowers our will and continues the habit and so we do it anyway which causes an uneasy confusion of the minds. The subconscious is a powerful force which makes it truly irresistible and a need to conform to the systematic habitual nature that has been learnt and developed over many years, hence the reason it is extremely difficult to kick the habit.

An often ridiculed form of therapy that can help shape and change pathways in our subconscious mind is hypnosis! Although viewed as a radical form of therapy with an air of mysticism about it and often met with a wall of scepticism, it is undoubtably an excellent therapy in the battle against any number of addictions because it directly taps into our hidden mind and alters specific imprinted habits and beliefs, which in turn changes the psyche and habit forming actions of everyday life. Although it has been gaining some popularity fleetingly in recent years, this practice has been proven not only effective in the pending fight against addiction, but also in changing the way we address phobias, unwanted psychological traits and much more.

We mentioned earlier how the subconscious mind is an emotional non logical mind and it takes in subliminally all that is around from the day we are born. It also takes care of all the automations we perform daily, from walking and riding a bike to driving a car. In these actions we rarely consciously make decisions, for if we did we wouldn't get very far as it is an extremely complicated process! We enter an Alpha mode, That's why (worryingly at times) on a motorway we might forget the last two junctions of our journey or ponder how we came to a destination so quickly. This mind also harbours the taught lessons and beliefs that have been passed down from outside sources and of course all of our habitual behaviours! Together with the fact it uses 90% of the brain's power it is no wonder we are so reliant upon it and why addictions are so hard to overcome. We will delve further into this topic later!

Maybe we escape for much shorter intervals. It could be something simple like a five minute break throughout the day for ourselves! Finding time to meditate, reading a few pages of our new favourite book, listening to music, these subtle practices can all help take life's stresses away, even if just momentarily. No matter what they are they all, in their own little way, help us face the rest of the day, But more to the point they help us to feel centred again, balanced and present.

Another escapism we all perform is daydreaming, this could be whilst taking a shower in the morning, cooking or tending to the ironing. When we daydream in these scenarios it is how we are feeling at that time which dictates the sentiment of the thought. If we are angsty or nervous of a pending meeting or even possibly telling someone unfavourable news and the like, when it comes to these specific thoughts we throw up a worst case scenario order of events, We do this to self-protect as anything other will be seen as a positive or bonus if you will, yet this only assists in making us go through the perceived stress of it all twice!

The last scenario is when we are in a calmer frame of mind maybe bored with our situation. Maybe the dreams and aspirations we longed for as children never fully materialised and so we start to dream big and wish for things in our head to escape the mundane reality of our existence. We might imagine we have won the lottery and are living in our mansion sipping champagne by our exotic poolside with our family and friends taken care of and enjoying life to the fullest! Then it dawns on us we haven't even had three numbers before! Or even won a crossword puzzle prize in the monthly magazine! Come to mention it we've never even worn a raffle at our child's school fair!

Then we are reminded of just how vast the odds of winning the lottery actually are. Referring to a mathematical theory we would have to play five lines twice a week for 81,000 years to stand against those odds! The UK National Lottery has odds of 1 in 45 million, The EuroMillions draw has odds of 1 in 139.8 million, And the Powerball In the USA has odds of 1 in 292 million and so we burst our own bubble with that dream!

So then we move on to slightly more realistic fantasies, Something we could possibly grasp with enough elbow grease and determination to reach that incandescent shimmering poolside, drinking our favourite bottle of fizz. You may or may not be accustomed to the new found belief in certain circles of social classes, that belief being The Secret! How to manifest your dreams into reality. With another dose of mysticism and no solid evidence many sceptics choose to see this train of thought as just slightly ludicrous, an intangible form of magic or figment of the imagination. We are bombarded with advertisements on social media and other search platforms on how to obtain it, the secret to bringing your deepest desires to fruition.

A simple subscription will be suffice, then you will be part of this inner sanctum and thus be able to create your own reality! Aren't you the lucky one to have stumbled upon such a charitable, genuine set of individuals? Willing to give you a way to realise your own dreams! Is this all just wishful thinking? At first glance is may seem so, the ironic part is the basic theory is correct, You see as we have just discussed with winning the ever-elusive lottery. One of the main advertising slogans is, 'You have to be in it to win It'. Now this is where the magic happens, just like the famous saying stipulates (although we will add an inclusion to lessen the bigoted tone) "They who think they can and they who think they cannot are both correct".

When we dream up such a life for ourselves and plant that seed deep inside our subconscious mind we also consciously give ourselves a direction to head in and a goal to strive for. Then as the quote delicately states, if we also have positive thoughts as opposed to the negative barriers we so often put up, we can start to see synchronicities develop which help reinforce this pertinent notion, and so our journey begins. It is not enough to merely think the positive thoughts. We also have to emotionally attach ourselves to this belief as we know the subconscious mind is an emotional mind and non-logical, therefore comparatively speaking we have to fake it till we make it!

This is quite important, you see, if you start to think you already have the life you wish to lead and embody it your mindset will also shift, giving and allowing yourself a rite of passage with a new found self-assured confidence. Then together with an awareness and living presently with our intentions and actions we invariably can and do create our own reality. There are many other factors that come into play when discovering or pursuing this topic.

What about the much more positive and beautiful aspects of escapism, namely the things we do for leisure. Not to discredit any other forms as they all assist, whether that be in a beneficial or unbeneficial type of way to our minds and bodies, they all in their own little way help us through the hardships we find ourselves in. But a real emphasis should be made when we refer to the more creative sides to escapism. As we all have a favourite hobby or pastime which we enjoy taking part in.

Let's look at that word 'pastime'. Why do we choose to participate in activities as a way of simply passing the time? Passing the time for what and to what end? Maybe they are just simple enjoyments to brighten our day or allow time to pass more efficiently until the next time we are truly enjoying ourselves. Our next vacation possibly! Yet it is much more than that! As we often see when we do partake in recreational activities we start to become passionate about these very things we initially viewed as just an simple interest. Of course a competitive streak can inevitably follow suit and we all know what the governing body is there! We can also single ourselves out as superstars for the talent we show and become admired by many for this. Who knows, possibly worldwide fame could be waiting in the wings!

When we are told to keep our feet firmly on the ground, to not get too carried away with ourselves, there is a common misconception apparent across the populace to a word we have all known throughout our lives. That word is 'nemesis'. Superheroes in comic books is the usual source in which we hear and learn this term, most if not all of the time it is used in conjunction with arch-rivals, the bad guy in the story, the true villain. The word 'nemesis' is derived from an ancient Greek goddess also called the goddess of

Rhamnous, who enacts retribution against those who succumb to hubris, a remorseless goddess that would show her treacherous wrath to any human who was arrogant to the gods.

In layman's terms she would relentlessly adjust the balance of human beings' actions in a karmic sense. She would reward those individuals who were humble, punish the evil, reward unacknowledged merit, deprive the worthless undeserved good fortune, chastise and humiliate the proud and overbearing (of which the ego is of profound importance here) and so maintain a righteous balance of things.

The reason for such fables from the ancient Greek culture was to instil certain beliefs in people - a necessity for a civilised existence. If you start to think you are a god in a sense, untouchable, then she will hastily cast you down from Olympus. We have all heard the saying, 'a fall from grace' or 'to be brought back down to earth'. We on occasions hypocritically like to also bring people back down to earth, dismounting them from their high horse! We take great pleasure in watching inflated egos falling from grace and can perform quite callous character assassinations, cutting them down to size at every opportunity but can soon feel sorry for them in their rapid demise.

Understandably this can be hard for such famed people to adapt to. How are they to stay grounded especially when they become idolised and are told just how great they are by the masses of adoring fans each and every day? Socrates proclaimed, 'fame is the perfume of heroic deeds'. This can be scaled down to all walks of life! When becoming a member of a team in our youth we will undoubtably come across a boastful character. With such terms as a 'glory hunter' being prominent and the spoken phrase, "there is no 'I' in team!" with the witty response, "No but there is a me in there somewhere".

When we start to elevate ourselves above those around us and begin to believe we are more important we have approached the message with a swing and a miss. We are that person next to us! Everyone working towards a common cause is undeniably more advantageous than trying to go it alone in every aspect of life! Team-mates may ridicule a member for performing badly instead of lifting them up. This is a much more positive action we should try emulate and embody in our daily lives with appreciation for just how fortunate our own circumstances actually are. Whatever the escapism may be, or whatever experiences they hold for all when we fall upon difficult times, remember the small things can make a difference, even the tiniest slither of excitement may be all it takes to get us through those tough situations, knowing that tomorrow is a new day full of possibilities with hope in our hearts as opposed to the lusts of desire is usually all that is required.

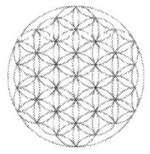

THE NEED

What are the fundamental needs of humanity from birth and for survival? Oxygen, sustenance, water and warmth. Any of these vital resources in high quantities can be of course dangerous so we will add enough! But they are essentially the basics for sustaining life. There is also procreation for the survival of the species but for now let us concentrate on the immediate factors Through the different classes into which we are born comes our sense of place in this social hierarchy, the existence or non-existence of wealth and status we find ourselves accustomed to can also bring with it a whole host of incredibly diverse psychological needs! The higher the class, the more the needs turn to desires, as opposed to the actual vitally important things our minds and bodies require in order to survive.

If we are born on the lower levels of this pyramid, the hopes and dreams are of the utmost basic; warmth, security, and just having enough food to get through the week. Plain survival! And so we become fixated on just that very primeval of instincts! Therefore our dreams and aspiration tend to take a backseat, the opportunities that are presented to people higher up are non-existent for the impoverished.

When we are busy with just trying to get by, the pipedreams become just that. How can we possibly think about becoming a talented musician, actor, actress, artist, scholar even the CEO of a bank, when we are caught in the doldrums? When just having a warm house and a belly full of food before sleep seems a dreamlike state. Yes as we have talked about, the many life lessons mould you into who you become, having nothing allows for a beautiful appreciation of the most fundamental attributes to life, and so when the lower classes do achieve their dreams it can stand them in good stead, for they understand what conspires to be, and their feet are planted firmly on the ground.

The only thing that can interfere with this is the tireless devil on the shoulder. This false higher sense of self tends to turn the underprivileged into the privileged, we have all heard the uttered phrase by the high achievers, "do you know who I am?". When faced with adversity, the wishes and wants we are told, we can achieve force us to work that bit harder so we may obtain such possessions, which also causes each of us to neglect some quite meaningful aspects to our life in the process.

We are also inundated by advertisements which target our imagined insecurities, they profess to know the very thing that will enrich our lives. Then the fear of missing out can soon become apparent, but all these so-called must-haves only have material value and will do nothing for our experience. They will only help people remain in the fallacy of popularity.

They say hard work is good for the soul but what is our interpretation of this? Work hard and you can achieve your goals, be mindful, do things presently, and gain that work life balance. The eternal need for wealth, status, acceptance, validation, instant gratification, is only followed by greed and corruption. True, we can achieve all of this and much more, but it has to be embarked upon with the right frame of mind, and without hurting ourselves or those around us in the process.

Wealth. Our perception of true wealth is mostly misguided. Take a trip to the local food store for instance, whilst grocery shopping more often than not we have begun to see this as a burden! The reason? Because we would much rather have and retain the monetary value as opposed to seeing the vital nutrients our bodies need for sustenance as the real wealth! But sadly in today's society we are so transfixed on digital figures we choose to see the numbers in our bank accounts as having the higher value.

Fame

There can be a need in a person for fame and stardom. This is a huge drive in today's culture, with the many inescapable technological platforms around each of us. Never has it been so effortless to achieve that five minutes of fame, the quintessential get rich quick scheme. The downside is that this sometimes hasn't been fully earnt and so without the full appreciation and hard work many don't acquire the illicit set of skills to handle and indeed navigate this fragile path. Fame is the ultimate carrot on a stick, due to the kudos and status that comes with such an achievement.

Some people's need for fame can be so overwhelming it can cause them to commit tremendous atrocities in order to answer that beckoning call of being known to the world, and fame quickly turns to infamy for these set of mentally deficient individuals. As their moral boundaries could be lacking considerably or completely erased from their minds, this dangerous mix is quite important when we talk about the need moving forward!

So why are we so highly driven in certain circumstances? it might not necessarily be for fame it might just be for a desirable career, to climb that mountain. You may just wish to test your physical human endurance, or in some cases you might wish to push your own faith to the limit with regards to extreme sports! Once again, intent has to be validated first, maybe reflecting upon why we have these insatiable desires at times should be addressed before we set off on the journey.

Reminding ourselves what we stand to gain and what we stand to lose. Many climb a mountain to find themselves and grow as a person as a result of the partaking. If your main objective from the things you do is to gain this experience then you are on the right path, but if it's to gain popularity or boost that false self then the issue lies solely at the love you have for yourself!

Learn to embrace the oddity that is you because, who wants to be a normal anyway? Start with absolute appreciation for your amazing peculiarities and depth of character for this is a great place to begin. Some people's needs and desires involve making a difference, or trying to change the world, yet can become fatefully misguided. Let's take medical science!

This scientific field has an unquenchable thirst for knowledge and is in a constant loop of trying to cure every illness and disease we find in the modern era. And because we appreciate this can help toward saving countless lives, needless pain and suffering for all, we doff our caps to this extraordinary science based research. But in recent years that hasn't been enough and now the focus is on preventing illnesses at a cellular level. Cloning, stem cell research amongst a multitude of other tests, trials and studies.

Big Pharma's gain is vast of course. If we can prevent a child from obtaining say sickle cell anaemia, leukaemia or non-Hodgkin's disease then of course we can all agree this is a worthwhile pursuit as everyone should at least be given enough of a life to enjoy and exist.

This topic is often pondered but fraught with controversy as we have to then look deeper! Do we try to prolong a life via any means possible? And to what end, Is it humane to do so? A violation of human rights? Maybe so, and is all conjecture, but what about locked in syndrome? Where it is the person affected who displays the determination? What existence are these unfortunate souls having?

This brings us onto the delicate taboo subject of euthanasia. Could euthanasia prevent the many cries for help with regards to suicide? As when we feel we are not forced back into a corner there can begin a prevailing sense of freedom and an awareness that we have been given a choice and a way out! This helps by instilling clarity of mind, and so the enormity of the thought can begin to lessen accordingly. So, can a law maker really have a right over the suffering of another? And should this be so? The opposing argument is that this direct source of suicide could give an option to those who may not be in the same category of suffering, namely those who are suffering in a depressive mental capacity. This then starts to become a trickier topic for that very reason, there is no unified, definitive answer as of yet. As this has been debated and debated in every court in every land with many differing outcomes and laws being passed. The whole euthanasia topic can cause conflict from every angle.

Peculiar things happen in life and yet there doesn't seem to be any rhyme or reason for it! Why can a person we deem unpleasant throughout their lives die of natural causes in their bed at the age of 89, yet a sweet innocent child die from a heart breaking illness at the age of 5?! When we are met by these types of circumstances we generally start to question our gods, our faith, even the universe or whatever we so believe - how is this right? How is this fair? What is the meaning behind such an act? Whether we are the metaphorical butterfly or tortoise in this life we all have to give it a certain level of meaning and credence regardless of the length, we have to just enjoy each moment and take just what we can from it.

The afterlife

The need to know what comes next! There are many theories to this! So, what happens to us after we pass? Is there a heaven? Is there hell? What is purgatory? Are we reincarnated? it all boils down to what we believe. If we believe we only get one shot at this thing we call existence then there will be much emphasis on death. We can't have a beginning without an end, right? But how can we then have an end without a beginning?

After all It is called the circle of life. Yet people associate this with the cycle of life and death, coming from the earth to go back to the earth, but what it actually represents is continuation. There is an instinctual need to survive and an overwhelming desire to live just that extra bit longer, yet how many of us actually live? Do we just find ourselves existing? Getting through to the weekend or reminding ourselves of that glorious holiday we have planned that's just round the corner? Are we just persistently trying to appease the fact we are stuck in our dead end jobs, with pressures of debt, burdens and responsibilities? Trying to survive the mundane boredom of everyday life? Can this force us to find a life worth living?

Large companies and indeed the government are highly adverse in the simple mind manipulation game, ever so slightly touching on triggers inside people that have a deep desire to be appreciated and liked by those that surround them. With today's generation of social media, technological chicanery. We get ourselves into tremendous amounts of debt and for what? Self-cynicism, as we are continuously told these very things will bring us joy, the business consortiums concoct a fictitious fantasy of how we ought to live with promises of gaining the good life. When we already know deep down the best things in life are free, the covetous nature of people, the need for flash cars, mansions, expensive luxuries, garish possessions, our wildest dreams, showing how cultured we are, these wants are all traits of insecure personalities. Overcompensation for the things we feel we lack. Not to say a beautiful home with all of its comforts won't enrich your life or the people close to you, just that we should carefully consider the reason and repercussions before diving into these things whole heartedly! A judgement call is often favourable in these circumstances. You work so hard and sacrifice so much to acquire this wealth and yet think nothing of those sacrifices when purchasing materialistic possessions to keep up appearances. Just ask yourself, do I actually need this? Will it ultimately serve me or is it just an ostentatious craving?

Branding has to be the greatest trick ever played on the unsuspecting public! Lead by trends and fashion, an inside joke by the big name brands to place labels on an items of clothing and popularise this fashionable attire. Yet many buy into these ludicrous ideas, can you see the humour in this and draw your own conclusion now? You see this hubris of the mind only keeps the rich, richer and endeavours to keep the poor, poorer, through the fear of becoming subjected to ridicule.

There is no need to try to make up for your imagined shortcomings or to win over people's hearts and minds, and so it should be the case of buying only the things that are going to make this experience as enjoyable as possible, and not for an envisaged acceptance.

If we stay on this hamster wheel of validation then that control over our lives that we tirelessly searched for can start to slip infinitely further from our reach. As for now yes we might feel trapped in our careers and start to become so resentful about the fact it plays absolutely no part in lifting our spirits, that it can start to feel like just a very simple necessity, and that dreamt up life and freedom we believed was our calling can become just an ambiguous train of thought.

Another common feature is the idea that we firmly accept the most appreciated normality to anyone's existence is to purchase a house and the endless years of juggling and struggling to pay for it! A small corner of this world to call our own, with the help of a friendly bank of course, who then proceeds to borrow you the funds via something called a 'mortgage' we then begin to tell all we know with such pride that "we have just bought our first home".

Let's just go back for a moment to that thing the bank very kindly offered so that we might be able to start our own little family in the comfort and security of a fixed premise. The word 'mortgage' is derived from the French words Mort and Gage meaning Death and Pledge as in the death of the agreement upon receiving funds in total.

The irony is that for many people the actual time it takes to pay back this amount can bring them precariously close to their own mortal fate, but regardless once we sign onto the dotted line we know ultimately that we will have to pay possibly 200% to 300% back over 25 to 30 years and so is the case, as to buy such an expensive commodity as a house outright to most is a ridiculous notion. Which is very true! unless we happen to obtain a windfall, the chances of us acquiring the house off our savings alone is slim to none, as to save that large sum of money we would have to be fortunate enough to have an understanding family who would be willing to let us stay in their home practically rent free for between 10 and 15 years. Usually what happens is, we try to save at least a sizable amount to put towards a deposit via this method of staying with parents or work every hour under the sun to save and gather enough funds together for the acquired total. So what is the answer? All of these things are the facts! The mortgage in principle is fine, it is the length of time it takes to pay it in full that can hold us back in so many other areas of our life, that is the issue! Also due to the fact that we are in this constant loop of trying to keep up appearances with lifestyle purchases we make we can end up needlessly extending this life sentence and the liberation we inherently crave can be left knocking. We are our own watchkeepers through the decisions we make daily, once you understand this and come to that realisation you will be given the key to the door and that sense of freedom will be yours. The ultimate dream is paying off our mortgage before we retire so that we can have a stress free retirement and also that there will be something left to pass on to our children, but the truth is most of the time that sum of money has to be divvied up into two, three or even four lots and is used predominately to pay off accrued debt the children have amassed up until that point.

We feel we can help facilitate a secure future for our nearest and dearest when we are not around, which is all well and good, the problem lies in how you view the mortgage! Many come to terms early on that it is just a formality at the end of every month and take no further credence to this, we carry on buying things we rarely need, we stay in jobs that begin to feel like a claustrophobic prison with no prospects of parole, we stop ourselves living a free life because of the sheer responsibility that comes with this persistent weight around our necks which year after year becomes heavier and heavier and can turn into our very own slipknot, an Atlas's burden if you will.

An answer could be as simple as sacrifice a little to gain a lot, restrain from the manipulation, start enjoying life for the things it presents to you freely and escape the talons of debt. Ask yourself this set of rhetorical questions, do I really enjoy the career I have chosen and are currently in? Have my youthful dreams been dashed? Is it ever too late to change? Are the responsibilities and burdens you currently face the main hold back or is it the fear of the unknown that prevents you from taking a leap of faith?

They say the best things in life are free, why is that? Let us list some of these things we might agree and deem to be the best things in life.

- Friendships.
- Love.
- Feeling happy.
- A good night's sleep.
- Helping others and the gratitude that comes with it.
- Watching a beautiful sunrise/sunset, nature's rolling landscapes.
- Looking up at the universal auditorium with its many flickering stars in the night sky.
- Being part of a family.
- Having a child.
- Humour.
- Feeling part of something.

This list is made up entirely of experiences and feelings. This is what makes life so special, these are the things that help us to feel alive and what stops us thinking we are merely existing. There are inherent instinctive needs that are hard to suppress as conscious beings, like the need and desire to procreate, to find a suitable partner with qualities that would offer our offspring the most beneficial start to life, from looks to physical attributes, predispositions to illnesses and disease, together with their personal ambition and moral persuasion. This is a self-protecting survival necessity at the basic level, the survival of the fittest gene pool, evolution, keeping the bloodline strong and long lasting.

We are running when we should be crawling in so many aspects of our lives in order to get to our goals at a faster pace, often losing who we are in the process and sacrificing our own beliefs and morals to obtain instant gratification, a reminder to people that everything is okay! So take one step at a time for you might fall over.

Also when we inevitably do make mistakes the point is not to try to correct our shortcomings but to be aware of them in the present. Most mistakes rectify themselves in time. If we try to right our wrongs we can sometimes swing this pendulum and exacerbate the impact! Trying to have dominion over it is a sure-fire way of magnifying any mistakes we make knowingly or unknowingly, often with the greatest will in the world and honest resolve. We have stark reminders of this scattered throughout the annals of history and even in the news and media today.

Wasted energy and futile pursuits

Let's use an analogy of the rower and the sailor. One uses tremendous effort in order to arrive at a destination, whilst the other gives his power away to nature and trusts in it completely. As the rower is busy tirelessly and methodically paddling their oars through the water sometimes against the current, they have no time or attention for the beauty around them. Yet the sailor who has efficiently harnessed the wind (which is causing the water to become choppy for the rower) to best effect. Not only that but they have also not wasted their energy unnecessarily and can appreciate the wonderous scenery, therefore being fully aware and present in the moment.

Now this is how we all can choose to live our own lives, the path of less resistance is always the most prosperous path of efficiency. If we are constantly in this fictitious battle to control all that is around or unwanted/unplanned blockades on the road to success we will invariably lose that vital energy to truly enjoy what greatness our life has in store for us, as this will only serve as a self-inflicted rigor mortis of soul. This isn't to say we should sit back in an idle pessimistic manner, it is merely to say that what will be will be! The rationale we choose will be the defining factor. The very thing that is meant for you will come to fruition regardless of any input, but knowing you are the universe and trying to stamp an egotistical will upon it is like trying to turn an apple into an orange or swim upstream when the current wants to take you down. When you don't oppose its force you will arrive at your destination with a comforting ease.

We should learn to enjoy each and every aspect whatever they may be, the good, the bad and the ugly for all the trials and tribulations are priceless commodities that teach us the very lessons we require as they are tests to help a person grow spiritually, guiding them on the rocky road ahead. So give away that power to the universe (as opposed to fighting it) and trust in it completely, only then will you start to see the flow of things, by embodying the Tao

(Pronunciation 'Dao') you will start to sense the many alignments happening all around and the perfect harmonious nature of the universe, therefore begin to move like water, and as you are not wasting energy on futile endeavours you can start to put that compassionate life force into great deeds. Yes, instantaneously an action will have an immediate reaction, as you can consciously say to yourself, "I will pick up that glass and take a drink of water" and the chances are you will. But now let's include a larger amount of time between the thought and the action, let's say you pick a time the very next day to perform the same task in the same place, would it be safe to say many other factors will start to come into play? Maybe a possible family emergency, an event at work, other commitments? Okay, we may be splitting hairs here, but it is still entirely possible to perform the said task.

Now let us stretch that time frame further to say a month. Will you even remember by then? Will your circumstances have changed? Are you sick in bed? On holiday or having a weekend away? Do you need to be at an appointment? The point of this is we can all have a will or a goal to head for, but the things that pop up out of our control need to be addressed in a positive way. We find ourselves from time to time saying, "isn't it funny how things work out for the best?" or "thank goodness we didn't do that". *C'est la vie*!

One path we choose could be an arduous one with lots of hurt, pain and hardships along the way, misspent youth or loss of precious time which could have been spent with our family and friends. When we begin to accept some of life's inevitabilities and start to use them to our advantage only then can we learn to enjoy this experience warts and all. Some people will try to counter argue this point by saying yes but what about in a crisis or medical emergency? Yes, that is true, some things require immediate action, the counterpoint being would most of these events have happened if the focus and momentary awareness was present? It is right, some things cannot wait for the great healer of time to play its role and if someone sees this as a valid point then they have mistaken the menu for the meal! The underlying message to this is when at times we consciously or unconsciously make a miscalculation regarding errors of judgement we all have an impending need to correct the mistake with a sense of urgency. But mostly this can be unwarranted if we just take the meaning from the lesson, and allow the self-induced drama to play out, then will we see that anxiety, self-doubt and negativity was the driving force of the outcome. What is fascinating is that more often than not, the outcome is only a fraction of the enormity we foretold in our minds.

Depravity

Depravity can lead to immediate irrational behaviour, as when we are deprived of oxygen our first instinct is to gasp for air. If someone is deprived of anything they instinctively need or desire for long periods of time they will act accordingly regardless of reason. Effectively taking what is not theirs in every conceivable aspect of existence imaginable.

The need to be liked

The need for popularity and a preferable public image (vanity) can go hand in hand in most cases, it is not solely for appreciation in the physical sense but how we are perceived by others from a characteristic standpoint. If people feel they need to be revered for their aesthetics then that person might be extremely inhibited and unhappy on the inside, so that is the issue and objective to be addressed firstly, a confidence boost from time to time by a friendly comment maybe just the ticket, but to constantly push ourselves to feel and appear as near to perfection as possible takes up a lot of time, not only that, but as a result we often attract likeminded people and these types of insecurities within a relationship can spread like a cancer.

To look handsome or pretty is fine and something we should all embrace, but when the time it takes to adorn this facade negates away from our life, we start to become a slave to our devilish entity. It causes a person to put on a false front physically and mentally. So just be you! And show up, remember, everything in moderation. It would be safe to say you and many of your close associates have missed out on great times for fear of not looking your best. Confidence is a preference. Own your positives and negatives but never stop living.

Do you feel there is a valid point to the fact that we/humanity become slaves to the idea that money brings happiness? What about the many get rich quick schemes, the much discussed pyramid schemes of life! Take the stock market for instance. Three things that will become apparent when delving into the treacherous world of the stock markets is manipulation, corruption and fear of missing out. The truth is we feel we can sway this action too, but on numerous occasions stock prices have gone up considerably on no news whilst other stocks have fallen sharply on positive news! It is all about sentiment!

A simple way to look at it is everyone puts money into a pot and a lucky few become very wealthy, on top of this the house takes a cut in the form of commissions, the government takes their 20% from any profits we accrue, (but turn the other cheek when we lose our house, their token gesture is that we may claim a loss in future years off our capital gains tax), also the companies and other unscrupulous characters manipulate the stocks all very underhandedly, but totally above board and legal in the eyes of the law, yet their acts cause fear and greed. Now with the use of diverse algorithms and faster internet speeds it can be akin to shooting fish in a barrel, we can also have dilution by unethical means.

Of course a few will profess to knowing the ins and outs and tell gleeful followers as to their next move allowing these wolves to exit profitable positions leaving the sheep carrying heavy bags, pump and dump marketed stocks cause a lot of unfortunate victims, the reason? Huge personal gain in next to no time. But as we all know the offset being huge personal lost, when we do not know the full extent to the workings of these markets we can stand to lose much more than our pride, so careful consideration has to be taken.

The truth of the matter is there has to be an influence, to what percentage? Nobody truly knows, but there are advantages when it comes to investing on the stock markets, as it can be likened to betting on a horse. You see you gain an insight and the ever so slightest control over the course as opposed to buying a lottery ticket, but that control is massively exaggerated in our minds. Not to say carefully considered investing will not pay off for you, it just takes us straight back to the theory that we should learn to crawl before we decide to run.

The need for power has always existed, for the past 10,000 years since early Sumerians existed between the Tigris and the Euphrates rivers and even before. Our many cultures and civilisations have always brought with them great (or not so great!) leaders. From then to now, kings, emperors, tsars, presidents, prime ministers and most notably fascist regimes brought on by dictators or tyrants depending on their tenure and degree of misuse of power. Some can be elected by the masses whilst others conquer with dominance to gain their seat at the top table. A better question is can we have a definitive in regards to when we rule or when we run a country? Is there even a dividing line? Power is said to change a person but this is not the case, it merely inflates our self-importance and magnifies our ego. The moment we feel we outshine our comrades is the moment our spirit is dwarfed by them, the more power we gain the harder it is to keep our feet on the ground and embrace spirituality. We think we can acquire both, but to gain one is to repel the other, we should never have a need or desire for power, as it serves us not.

We can get so overwhelmed at times with the deep desires within us that they become near impossible to resist, the temptation factor! As long as the aim is just, it should not be resisted or revoked. Everything can start to become personal to each of us no matter what the subject, we find ourselves wanting to be noticed and listened to, we cannot help but voice our opinions onto others. Rarely, though, do we listen and respect other people's points of view. How many times have you found yourself in a one-way conversation? Or have you ever feigned interest in another person's likes so that you too may be liked by that same person? Something strange seems to happen to all of us, we feel terribly uneasy when somebody else takes a disliking to us. We start to doubt ourselves, but also question the other person, as we must try to command this situation and sway their inclination in our direction. Once again, power, control, confidence and pride all come into it, but the strangest thing comes about when you take no interest in their preference or even that person. They start to become intrigued by you, and curiosity wins out. They begin to question why you are not taking any notice of them and start to be drawn ever closer to you in a sort of subtle admirable type of way.

So, what is the message we can attain from this? When we force things we can end up pushing them further away! So, turn away from negativity and see what magnificence this world has in store. We begin to attract positivity without any effort! Many have this constant requirement to be adored by all, but that is just a hopeless dream, for although it is nice to have pleasantries passed onto us by a lot people, it is the people who challenge us that brings about biggest spiritual growth and for that we should be grateful. Show your value, show your worth, show self-appreciation not self-obsession because let's face it that only leads to self-criticism, mental anguish and death by a thousand cuts.

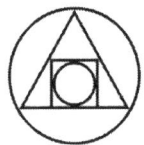

PHILOSOPHY

Philosophy is the study of the fundamental nature of knowledge, reality and existence. It can also be a theory or attitude to live by subjectively. For eons we have asked ourselves the existential questions, why are we here? For what purpose? What is the meaning of life? To look at the stars and look deep inside our souls unshakeably knowing that there is more to life than we are currently aware of. If this is your take on things then you are firmly in the Existentialist's camp. Whilst if you believe life is just life with no further meaning and once you pass you are all but worm's meat then you embody that of a Nihilist. There are different variations to each. We also have the Absurdists, for example, whose philosophy is based on the belief that the universe is irrational and meaningless and that the search for order brings the individual into conflict with the universe and their own mind.

Let's imagine we are back in ancient Greece sitting in the gallery listening to the likes of Socrates and his student Plato and slightly later on in this era, Aristotle! Would we agree with the theories they present? Or would they be too far removed from our ways of thinking? Culturally and generationally, possibly, as the way we think and interpret theories is all relative to our environment and the times in which we exist. This all has an impact on how we process these thoughts. Let's take out what we can from the many quotes and theories and try to understand the main premise to each and what is relative to our own times.

Academics have a clear definitive meaning behind each quote, but you can have your own interpretation and that may prove to be the most beneficial to you and yours. Putting your own spin on things will ultimately help you to understand the philosophy behind the quotes from a personal perspective with much more poignancy, which in turn will serve as a more meaningful and relevant idea to yourself. We can all peruse the internet for the meanings of famously profound quotes but are sometimes met with sterile paragraphs of subjective meanings from lectured citations. So now let's try to digress through a few different quotes by many a famous philosopher and as we do ask yourself do you agree! Or better still create and find your own powerful meaning?

Past philosophers and a slice of their work

Socrates

"True knowledge exists in knowing that you know nothing." Meaning? What can we extrapolate from this? Possibly what he is trying to put across is that knowing that there are things in existence out of the realms of man and though we cannot see such things, therefore not understand their true nature, being aware of the possibilities may be in itself knowledge.

"An unexamined life is not worth living." If our life is a tree of fruitless endeavours is it worth living? And so not to reflect on the good or bad memories, our joys our regrets is to not have lived a life at all.

Plato

"The punishments which the wise suffer who refused to take part in government is to live under the government of worst men." In today's society the simplest meaning could be, if as wise citizens we don't take an avid interest in politics and our own governmental rule, and subsequently not cast our own vote we will invariably be ruled by lesser people full of corruption and morally objectional ambition and as a result not be able to have a voice in this matter.

"Courage is knowing what not to fear." The aspect of this quote is twofold: it states that having knowledge of what to fear and what not to fear therein lies the truth, that judgement of what is good for us and what is bad for us, only then can we learn the virtues and embrace life fully.

"There are two things a person should never be angry at, what they can help and what they cannot." The actions we take in our lives are explicitly linked to our individual choices and the universal elements of existence, and so to be angry at such things can make no sense. Also, on the other side of this coin, how can we possibly show vexed sentiments at occurrences which are out of our control?

Aristotle

"Suffering becomes beautiful when anyone bears great calamities with cheerfulness, not through insensibility but through greatness of mind." We can choose to give ourselves completely to suffering, for in the act of giving the power away is what also makes us powerful! We should see the lesson from the suffering and not treat it with contempt, but with a wry smile for then can we see it as our teacher and watch to see for the message and so to witness this act by someone with a steely smile, although harrowing, can leave a profoundly beautiful image in our mind.

"He who cannot be a good follower, cannot be a good leader." This is quite self-explanatory but nonetheless shows much relevance in our generation. It has an underlying hypocritical tone, how can we expect others to follow us when we cannot follow others? To lead by example could be deemed a modern reiteration of this term.

"Men acquire a particular quality by constantly acting in a particular way." As we have discussed, we are habitual creatures, this is the learnt behaviour strategy our subconscious mind perpetuates. Habits are hard to break, this is also how we can categorise people in our lives. Some people may like solitude and abstain from social gatherings so we may call them a loner. Someone who has a humdrum affinity with life could be seen by others as a miser. We can and often do pigeonhole many from different walks of life by their quirks and traits. If you persistently do something you will soon get noticed for it thus forming the character as seen by others, it becomes the fabric in which we are perceived by those around us.

Now let us look at quotes from the modern philosophers of the past few centuries and how we may interpret their ideas, from the likes of Nietzsche right through to Descartes.

Friedrich Nietzsche

"Blessed are the forgetful for they get the better even of the blunders." Essentially, ignorance is bliss is a simpler way of putting it, but without the body and depth. We are all aware of our actions at times and the impact it can have on others and sometimes some amongst us are fully aware of the downsides to others by their actions but continue forth regardless.

"He who has a why to live can bear almost any how." They who can find a purpose to their lives with positivity and a direction to head for can push past any hurdle or obstacles in the way, once you find the reason to live, the how's of life become of no concern.

"To live is to suffer to survive is to find some meaning in the suffering." There have been numerous interpretations of this as with most philosophical excerpts, through life we suffer, we fight to survive every single day, to give life meaning and a reason is also to give meaning to the suffering.

Soren Kierkegaard

"Life is not a problem to be solved but a reality to be experienced." This also is quite transparent. It is merely advice to be taken, a gentle nudge, we should not see life or approach life perpetually thinking of solutions to problems we should just live the experience laid before us. We can get too hung up on the negatives instead of cherishing the positives! Any fly in the ointment should be seen as just that, part of the process.

"Boredom is the root of all evil." The despairing refusal to be oneself. The most meaningful one of recent times, the devil makes work for idle hands to do. We are so used to audible and visual stimuli we become irritably bored when we are caught alone with our thoughts, we have a responsibility to ourselves to learn how to be alone as only then can we discover who we truly are.

"Don't forget to love yourself." Another gentle reminder we get so caught up in loving others and things we very much neglect ourselves in the process, we can and do interpret this as being selfish which couldn't be further from the truth! We have to stop feeling guilty for who we are and learn to love thy very nature and so essence of our true self.

Rene Descartes

"If you would be a real seeker after truth, it is necessary that at least once in your life you doubt as far as possible all things." Take nothing for granted we have to be able to question everything as to not broach things in a naive way, for the fact we can question existence is the very thing that also makes it real! To be able to conceivably doubt things is to be able to think the thought and so start to formulate an answer to life.

"Except our own thoughts there is nothing absolutely in our power." This has a stoic undertone, one that has had big thinkers at loggerheads for some time. Some agree with this, many oppose it, here's why. He's trying to say everything external is outside of our control, only the mind/our thoughts is within our control, many would argue that not even our thoughts are totally within our control, as when one tries to think of nothing they begin to think of everything.

"In order to improve our mind, we ought less to learn, than to contemplate." We can all learn knowledge in a parrot fashion style and sometimes most of that information is lost to memory if we don't use that knowledge in our daily lives, and so we end up overwriting the information with much more recent meaningful statistics. It would therefore serve more purpose to learn a small amount intimately and reflect upon it and try to understand it in its entirety.

Immanuel Kant

"Live your life as though your every act were to become a universal law." This is a morally centred excerpt, a "do unto to others, as you would want done unto you" as it would be hypocritically condescending to treat others and life with contempt but still expect the best from them in return. Use your own moral compass to navigate this journey, what you deem righteous is what you should embody in this life.

"All our knowledge begins with the senses, proceeds then to the understanding, and ends with reason, there's nothing higher than reason." To know firstly has to be seen, felt, heard, witnessed. Only then can the information arrive in our minds, we then try to conceptualise this information and understand its meaning, what is the root of this, and lastly we reason with it, this is to say, do we agree with this non judgementally? For only then can we fully take it as read or as black and white as a fact.

Jean-Paul Sartre

"Man is condemned to be free, because once thrown into the world he is responsible for everything he does." Dictators, tyrants with no guide seem to act on devilish intent, We have to own our actions rightly or wrongly, therefore stand by our convictions even when condemned by them. It is down to us as individuals to be responsible for what we do for better or for worse, and this to Sartre was a frightful concept, as if we were ruled by a tyrant the book would lie solely with them.

"When the rich wage war it is the poor who die." This is an immensely powerful notion for current affairs of the recent decades, the world leaders plan strategies sometimes for unethical reasons pertaining to war, sometimes for greed sometimes for power, they are so far removed from the battlefield of young souls they cannot and do not dwell on the consequences of the decisions.

"If you are lonely when you are alone then you are in bad company." This above all is the most powerful of quotes. When considering ourselves as the third person would you be with someone who put you down all the time? Would you become bored with the incessant negative talk? Would you be spending your quality time with someone who did not excite you? To feel alone in your own company, is not to know thyself.

"Everything has been figured out except how to live." This is similar and on the same lines as Kierkegaard's, "life is not a problem to be solved but a reality to be experienced." We try so hard to figure all the things that make up this universe that we forget to exist, at times we should just be with a quiet contentment.

We can all be considered philosophers, having our own take on the interpretations of life and the meanings behind them, as through our life we begin to form different perspectives.

Do we romanticise about such theses from times gone by? Say if someone in our times had been the first to pen such theories would they have the same profoundness as how we think of quotes from our forefathers? Undoubtedly these scholars were of the utmost intelligence and it would be fair to say far ahead of their time. Socrates for one had a real problem with the democratic system of the Athens Government and opposed it at every turn, openly objecting to it throughout his life. His reasoning was that he believed only philosophers had the credentials to suitably govern others. He also pointed out that human choice was motivated by the desire for happiness and so wanted to establish an ethical system based on human reason rather than theological doctrine.

The problem philosophy has is that most of it is subjectively thought and written, it can be biased and opinionated, we can all have our own opinions and beliefs but we can't have an opinion that opposes a fact. As humans, we will always try to seek the truth and when that cannot be obtained we counter argue a point to try to whittle it down to the most probable. Often we stand for an argument that we don't fully believe in just to push the opposition into a corner as a way of poking and prodding them into giving us more substance to their theory and so giving us the most likely of possibilities, this unwavering compulsion for truth, for concrete proof, for the irrefutable facts. We can't simply allow ourselves to believe in something intangible without hard evidence.

In scientific terms the quantum realm or even in the field of astrology the facts we have presented to us today may be so far from the truth in years to come we will wonder how we ever bought into such things, as in yesteryear we firmly believed that the sun revolved around the earth and that the earth was the centre of the universe! Now with advanced technology we know that not to be true, many incredible leaders in their specific fields have theories accepted by their peers as fact or most probable to have it disputed later on in time or found to be inaccurate.

The point to this is that what you have been taught through your life whether you are consciously or unconsciously aware of it, may not necessarily be correct, and if we hold on to these beliefs and not allow ourselves to be open enough to the alternatives then we cannot evolve mindfully. On the flip side, if something you believe in gives you hope or helps you through your life it cannot be discredited. Don't allow others to influence or sway you into taking a more accepted, popular notion, if it comes from within, allow it to reside there.

INDIVIDUALITY AND CREATIVITY

Individuality, the uniqueness and character of a particular person, the separate existence. We often think it is our will and oneness that forms our own individuality and possibly this may be true to a certain degree. An eclectic mix of personal preferences and amalgamations of the visual, audible and conceptual, we seem to take titbits of information and aesthetics and fashion them into our own vision.

We have established that character is thrust upon us from many different sources, we are also aware of the fact that we are taught to believe certain truths from an early age. Also we are constantly in a submissive state from the authoritarian life teachers, together with bodily developments rapidly changing our anatomy throughout the pubescence stage. It is not surprising then, that we start to develop this overwhelming need to carve out a niche of our very own from this world of dominance. This in turn causes our rebellious streak where we may start to put our idiosyncratic stamp on who we are. Anything from a style of clothing, getting a piercing, a tattoo, dying our hair, having a unique hairstyle, being drawn to a certain genre of music, the social group we take, the list is endless. From a whole manner of things, this allows a person to transition from the naive to the responsible, which sounds counter intuitive to say that as an outcome to a rebellious spell, but the premise being it can help us to find our place in this world. But in doing so we lose a lot of our wonderment and awe for life. It is an absolute necessity to allow this, as parents or guardians, to occur naturally without an impairment of any kind, unless of course the actions become unlawful or perilous. For if we choose a path of discipline this can instil the evocative connotations that undoubtably come with such a method, and so we should (even against our better judgement) permit this transitional period.

We all have to just trust, reason and empathise otherwise we can act as two identical poles of a magnet, and unintentionally become the object of power they so oppose, so when the time comes for them to seek guidance they will feel they have alienated themselves, and in their time of need will try to go it alone and subsequently end up lost navigating this often beautiful but sometimes treacherous world.

At every turn on this journey our persistent friend whispers to us, "you are different" "you are special" "you are unique" "so let the world know this". So you strive to be! The persistent sprite is perfectly correct nonetheless! You are special! You are different! You are extremely unique! But it is the ambition that is implied by our friend on the shoulder that causes misguidance, physically, characteristically and spiritually you are undeniably one of a kind! But you are also it, the Tao! You come from the same thing we all come from and you share the same collective consciousness of all. The persistent mind chatter irrevocably forces you to become different, to go against the grain, when all that was needed was for you to just be you.

Being unique has given rise to many beneficial feats for mankind, there have walked countless brilliantly minded people on this earth, who have all created distinctive masterpieces, from colossal problem solving, incredible inventions to cultural advances, and still do to this day. We will mention just a few of these amazingly creative ideas and see how they have benefited humanity and we as individuals in our daily lives, and question if any have stayed true to their purpose or if they have been adapted to be used against our species and indeed the planet.

Let's begin with inventions, from the invention of the wheel to the microchip, from a flint arrow head to the MRI scanner, each is perceived as a human and cultural advancement which is a positive note that cannot be argued with. The negative side is that as a race of beings we will continue to search indefinitely for bigger and better, partly down the wrong path in some cases! We are told to roll with the times and yes we should be flexible to adapt to change, the whole evolution of things, which we question so often. But to do so we have to also question the need and what might be the negative impacts to each, so the main question is, is it a real problem or is it an inconvenience? The patent office's floor is scattered with dreams and fruitless studies that may have helped clean up a lot of humanity's historical wrongdoing to the environment, but were seen as non-profitable ventures. Yet many seemingly impractical inventions that serve no great purpose have been put forth to the world due to consumerism, sometimes a reflection of the greater good ought to be the main focus not profit, that is the pressing issue.

A list of human concepts and their coming to be is thus: scientific works, construction, medical advances, literature, language, art, astrology, quantum physics, architecture, government, mathematics, technology, numerous problem-solving notions for instance genetically modified crop developments, famine and water shortages solutions, environmental factors, namely climate change and carbon foot printing.

The ever-present balance of things, what have been the good and the bad to come out of such inventions, do they still get used today for their intended use? For the most part yes, but there are some exceptions. We will touch on a few significant inventions plucked out of the history books from the earliest forms to the present.

Let us firstly take a look at one of the earliest cultural inventions, fire. Also argued this is a natural occurrence merely observed by early man therefore not an invention, but the act in which it was harnessed and made was of course a hugely beneficial advancement for human civilization. This very act created by humans sought to become a comforter for warmth and protector against the elements, of wild beast and of other humans. The most powerful of impacts was the ability to cook sustenance and so obtain higher nutritional value, which in turn allowed an evolution, advancement and expansion of our brain structure to happen. This over millennia gave birth to early forms of civilisation.   It also may have helped   our predecessors gain the upper hand against relative species namely (homo neanderthalensis), also the use of tools by early humans, from flint arrowheads, spears and cutting blades. These useful commodities combined also helped further the evolution of homo sapiens, as this allowed our species to become much more effective and efficient hunter gatherers with a secondary bonus of serving to protect against the many predators in the Middle Palaeolithic period.

Now let's move on and delve into the exploitive depths of humanistic inventions, boat making, ship building, the use of compasses and telescopes, trains, cars, aeroplanes, steam engines, spaceships, our advancement in travel and our unquenchable thirst to explore our environment and search for new horizons, which can also hold the key to answering such questions as, where do we come from? And how did we come to be? We now have (in the development stages) a manned mission to Mars, possibly to colonise the red planet in the future, therefore making it habitable.

Boat building, it is theorised that due to archaeological studies and data, homo erectus may have crossed bodies of water to new landmasses hundreds of thousands of years ago, on what? Well this is up for speculation; whatever it be, it could still be categorised as a vessel of sorts in a primitive sense. A reed bed, palm fibres binding sections of bamboo together, a fallen trunk (dugout) the reason is also up for debate. A pure series of coincidences, storms, to explore, for survival, endless possibilities. Indigenous people were said to have inhabited Australia as far back as 50,000 years ago crossing vast stretches of water to arrive at the shore of this new exotic land.

The earliest forms discovered date back roughly 12,000 years, the 10 foot Passé canoe being the oldest manmade boat unearthed, and so through the years with needs for development the materials and tools fashioned to create such crafts had to be perfected, along with the shape and design so that it could become significantly more structurally sound, allowing for greater capacity and speed. Regardless, it would be a fair assumption that the initial incentives would have predominantly been that of an explorative one or possibly a primitive matter of survival, and so a way to gain nourishment from the sea. We have to now see if the same pure incentives remained throughout our history, cut to ancient Greece and the battle of Salamis. Whilst King Leonidas was taking on the might of the Persian army, as his last stand against King Xerxes was being written into the history books at Thermopylae, there was a Navy battle also taking place just off the coast of Salamis between the alliances of the Greek city states under the command of the Athenian Themistocles and the immensely powerful Persian Navy.

We start to see subtle hints of how something of pure intent can start to be used for a less than favourable cause, the balance of good and bad, of course these wars between two factions would have inevitably occurred, as it has for millennia on land driven by greed and the need for power, to conquer all. On the Greek side the vessels were used to optimum effect against the tyrant's navy and freedom prevailed after the slaughter, but it just emphasises our need for technological enhancement, as through the ages it can and has been used for lesser good or in assisting in our demise and will continue to do so unless we rationalise the outcome prior and learn to hold onto that thought when coming up with such ideas. Is there a really a prevailing need? What are the downsides/repercussions? With honest foresight ask, how can this be used and turned against humanity? If our self-importance wasn't so much of a gigantic presence in the world today this specific set of questions would fall principally redundant, and so in the future these very puzzlements would be of certain irrelevance. The Viking hordes crossing the North Sea to find new fertile pastures to use in agriculture soon turned into a more sinister expedition of rape, pillage and conquer, wiping out villages and to some extent spreading disease not of the land. Now we turn to aviation. Our longed for quest to be able to soar through the clouds as free as a bird. An amazing achievement yet it only took 11 years from the invention of the first plane by the Wright brothers in 1903 to its use in its first battle during WW1 where it had been adapted to facilitate the dropping of bombs and taking with it many innocent lives.

Fast forward 30 years to Enola Gay and the dropping of the first Atomic bomb in 1945. Many proclaim ending WW2 although there were many factors that lead to this, the two United States nuclear bombs were detonated on the Japanese cities of Nagasaki and Hiroshima which resulted in the death of over 130,000 people, mainly innocent civilians, and injuring countless more in one fell swoop.

Today we have unmanned aircrafts called AVEs navigated by a ground based controller, comparable to a computer simulation game, which can leave devastation and destruction in its wake on any mission. The progressive nature is plain to see. Now we will move on to the scientific world of medicine, one of the most amazing and prominent medicines that first comes to mind is Alexander Fleming's incredible discovery of penicillin. This specific drug has saved millions of lives and also millions of people from pain and suffering. Its origin and discovery is a peculiar story to say the least. Whilst researching and experimenting with the influenza virus in the laboratory of the inoculation department at St Mary's Hospital in London he was also experimenting with other pathogens and bacterium.

One such common bacteria staphylococcus (which can have huge health implications on patients with weakened immune systems) had been carelessly left exposed on a culture plate. Also strange was that somebody had left a bowl of broth close to its proximity.

Upon his return to the lab after holidaying for two weeks, Fleming made a startling discovery. He found that a mould had developed, accidentally contaminated the staphylococcus culture plate, and on further examination of the mould he noticed that the strain of mould had prevented the growth of the Staphylococci. He stated, "Staphylococcus colonies became transparent obviously undergoing lysis, the process in which mould had been grown, hardening temperature for one to two weeks had acquired marked inhibitory, bactericidal and bacteriolytic properties to many of the more common pathogenic bacteria." You see a somewhat strange and accidental series of events led to one of humanity's greatest cures! And yet we put it down to a mere coincidence with a positive outcome, without contemplating it further but just with a debt of gratitude to the discoverer.

The steam engine and the birth of the industrial revolution. The first pattern for a steam engine was made by Thomas Savery In London in the year 1698 which he referred to as the miner's friend, since its intended use was to pump water from the mines. Early versions left much to be desired as the soldered copper boilers would rupture upon even low steam pressures. With careful tweaking and redesigning throughout the years a much more robust and powerful steam engine was created, this in turn gave a kick start to what we know now and refer to as the Industrial Revolution! Between 1760 and 1840 took place a distinct transition to a new and far more efficient manufacturing process in Europe and the United States. This shifted the manufacturing of goods from small shops and work houses to large factories, it also had a huge effect on our culture as people started to move from rural areas to big cities in order to find better paying jobs. The steam engine was utilised to power these colossal processes, allowing for a more productive and cost effective solution.

The health implications to the workers in these tight-knit communities surrounding such industries was detrimental to say the least. We have all seen images from the remnants of this era, black and white photographs of chimney stacks, narrow street dwellings and plumes of smoke in the air. Like with anything the industrial living areas soon became cramped and squalor began to exude from the despot side streets where poverty rang out from every corner, people often found themselves destitute in quite bleak conditions where their only salvation came in the premise that hope was left residing in the box. If you were unfortunate to lose your job through a dispute at work or became lame through old age or even due to a work related accident and deemed worthless by the factory you then had to muster all you could to gather together enough coppers to gain adequate sleeping accommodation from a lodging house by any means possible. Or if you fell short of the fee you had the option to pay tuppence to sleep under a roof on a rope with a watch man standing lookout (which illustrates our complex adaptabilities perfectly) this is where we get the term, 'you could sleep on a washing line'. Because of the sheer scale of the operations many unscrupulous characters were able to amass vast wealth and status. Although an incredibly intelligent and savvy business minded approach, the morality was inherently lacking, with child labour, untold injuries and deaths the actual health of the workers would play a firm second fiddle to profits and a third would come the environment.

This thirst for success and production has never really wavered since that time. It has only served to become a measurement in which to achieve greater things, bigger is better! An incredible fact to illustrate just what impact the industrial revolution has had on humanity and the life we lead today is, it took 200,000 years of human existence to reach a billion in global population, circa 1804, but it took less than 200 years to reach 7 billion, circa 1999, an astonishing increase by a factor of 7! Better sanitary conditions, higher paying jobs, better housing, advancements in healthcare are all contributing factors.

The average age of death in 1804 was a mere 49! Now with a global population of 7.7 billion the average

age of death is 82.9, an increase of roughly 60% and predictions for 2100 is a world population of 10.9 billion. This might cause some economic problems of its own, also food shortages, and the destruction of nature for habitation. This process cannot be stopped. Maybe it is meant to be, but we have to account for that now and not then! The untold harm we have caused our planets in the last 200 to 300 years is evident, big steps are being made to rectify some of the issues, but what it all boils down to, is our lower self instilling a self-righteous need that was never called for. Of course we must move with the times otherwise we may get left behind, but it is up to the global population as a community to create those very times, as a collective conscious, than to idle away any hope.

Most inventions today are there to make one's life easier, but we have to ask what are we losing or giving away as commutation? Take an important one of the times, the smartphone! It seems this device can completely organise our life making almost any task seem like a breeze, with the abundance of apps and the various ways to communicate it would appear that many people in the first world could not be without this amazing creation. Any answer to any question is all but a finger press away. A person with knowledge but with no understanding is usually a dangerous mix, mind you. It is irrefutable that this technology is nothing short of incredible, it is in the way in which we use this technology that could be the defining factor! This small but powerful invention has opened up the entire world to us all, it has helped people connect with friends, family and past acquaintances, but through the ever present popularity quest it can also connect them to a whole populace of people they may not necessarily cross the street to say hello to! The most negative impact social media has is how it can force people to compare their lives to others and as a result become self-critical or worse, fall into a pit of depression and anxiety. "What one hand giveth the other taketh away."

Inevitably, there will be a presence of bullying on such sites just as there is in life generally, or overly opinionated people craving acceptance. But one of the main factors to the negatives that reside on social media is the comparable aspects. You see when we, like with drugs, become addicted to browsing these domains something that started off as a pastime to stave off the monotony and boredom of daily life, turns quickly into an absolute necessity and so we begin relentlessly perusing the inescapable social network. This quickly changes our demeanour! We start to become more and more aware of other people's lives, achievements, celebrations, new life, new partners, new babies, new house, a steady flow of fortunate circumstances. This causes much anguish and serves as an unwarranted yardstick upon which we start questioning our own life and the why's and where's start formulating around our heads!

Why have we not got the career we wanted? Why are we single? Why are we renting a house? The why is irrelevant, as what is meant for you will come to light regardless of intent. The flow has no time frame just a will. If we try to dictate this and allow frustrations to take over we will drive it further from our life. If we allow it to synchronise and develop naturally we will start to see small yet meaningful events transpire before our very eyes.

One point to contemplate is, if when we are glued to a screen for hours a day, are we essentially trying to live our lives in an imaginary flotation tank? A total recall of sorts? If you were given the option to enter such a tank for the remainder of your life, programmed for you to live out your deepest desires as if it was as real as your reality now, would you choose to opt out of your life and enter into this fantasy with what you know now? Many have pondered this question however, the answer you give may just reveal a hidden message.

Our problem-solving techniques have at times paid dividends, monumental construction dilemmas, water and food shortages, medical advancements, sanitation, environmental factors. But the most beautiful and pertinent aspects to creativity comes in the forms of the muses, most notably music, art and literature, you see when it comes to this type of creativity it is in the doing where we get the most joy, not necessarily the final product. When in connection with ourselves and the universe we enter a tranquil flow state, this enables a person to dance the dance and become their true self, allowing for great masterpieces to flow and fall onto the parchment in front of their very eyes. When we paint, it is not just the final brush stroke that is the important aspect but the actual act and journey that is developed which is the most pleasurable part. When we play music, our aim isn't to get to the last note, it is in the playing we take the most joy. When writing or reading a book it is the story, the evocative notions that compels us to carry on, placing ourselves inside that world with ardour for more. This is the wonderment not the final outcome. We sometimes hope and pray for it to finish on a cliff-hanger, an open ended finale, with the reassurance of a sequel, this is a perfect analogy to our own journey, the ending isn't the most prevalent part! It is the magnificent adventure in which we should gain the most!

Not trying to go as fast as we can to the finish line, constantly living our thoughts in the future, we have to stop and appreciate the importance of now! The moment you are reading this is the only moment there is, and just like that, that moment has passed. The future you try so hard to imagine and control is an illusion, a fallacy, a fictional tale you tell yourself. You have to be able to smell the smells, see the sights, and hear the sounds all around.

Art

What images come to mind when you think of art? Possibly Leonardo da Vinci's Mona Lisa? Michelangelo's David, the beautiful renaissance sculpture? Damien Hirst's amazing centrepiece, the physical impossibility of death in the mind of someone living? Or is your consciousness drawn more to the performing arts side of things? Whatever your preference it goes without saying art can embody a wealth of emotions deep inside. Art has a way of speaking to us all without saying a word, it can be provocative, have elements of sadness, have a spiritual origin, it can make us happy, help us put things into perspective, but above all else it helps us to be in the moment. When we are observing a piece of art in any form we stop wholeheartedly and gaze deep inside. The background audio and shadows in our peripheral vision all but disappear, we become transfixed trying to fathom the true meaning of the works or trying hard to find out what drove the artists to create such enigmas.

Literature

Similarly the written word has the same powerful impact on humanity. When we read powerfully stunning novels by the likes of Charles Dickens, Jane Austen, George Orwell, Roald Dahl and JK Rowling to name but a few, we become engrossed by each chapter, imagining we are the main character and feel every sensation alongside them, fully encapsulated by the storyline. The evocative nature causes sensitive feelings to be triggered by each sentence of the dialogue. For this very reason it becomes apparent we give ourselves completely to this imaginary realm and get sentimentally attached to the work. It helps broaden our mind, see circumstances from a different point of view, see the bigger picture! It also can force us to empathise with the thoughts of menacing characters and take them in as our own, compartmentalising the acts they had previously committed. We become fully immersed in the book, totally lost and absorbed in each thread - a joyous time of relaxation beside a log fire in the depths of winter with our favourite tale conjures up comfortable warming images inside our minds. Then of course not to forget the many incredible poetry works we have had left by the likes of T.S. Eliot, Emily Dickinson, Dylan Thomas and William Wordsworth! and they are just a small drop in the ocean when it comes to the astonishing depth of poetry works left to us today.

Poetry has a profound nature, whilst intelligently written, most are often short and yet say so much without saying very much at all. It is thought provoking, evocative, can touch our souls and give meaning to thoughts we have momentarily wondered.

When all is said and done literary works paint pictures without the use of a single brush stroke, and that in itself is a joy to behold.

Music

The dictionary description for music is 'vocal or instrumental sounds combined in such a way as to produce beauty of form, harmony and expression of emotions'. Music can be lyrical works of art, that appears to recite a message relating directly towards our own existence, therefore we can begin to identify unconditionally with that song's meaning, it can also light a fire from deep within. We all gravitate towards a certain genre of music which forms parts of our character. We all have guilty pleasures we keep to ourselves. A particular song can bring up the evocative emotion of nostalgia, be filled with sadness or joy and help us to get through a particularly turbulent breakup. When we hear an upbeat song playing the fast tempo forcefully compels our personalities to become more energetic. Our subconscious mind interprets this in a nanosecond and the conscious mind feels the sensation soon after, and with the already feel good hormones racing around our bodies the intoxicating thrill of life can rush over us, causing bodily movements sometimes out of our control. It might be a simple foot tap, a head bop or a hand motion, whatever it is, dance is soon inevitable. Our emotional response to the vibe! When our ear drums are stimulated by the pulsing beat it can sometimes bring about such an immense feeling that we become lost, saturated by a wave of euphoria. Do you ever find that a song you didn't much care for in your youth played by your parents now becomes a treasured memory when caught off guard by it in adulthood? It too, as well as art, communicates to our higher self. This is enhanced further by the frequency and vibrations as they permeate deep inside. You could say when music is played it is the soul that sings!

The performing arts

Whether it be drama, theatre, film, ballet, magic, comedy, the performing arts can be awe inspiring. It helps spread a message, gives life to relevant topics of the times, it can educate and provoke a person into action. But what it does so importantly is it engages with people, it makes them sit up straight and observe with its elements of mystery by its intelligent use of smoke and mirrors, it has a way of capturing our imagination, it has substance we can relate to with subject matters of lust, greed, power, love and sadness.

With an opening which more often than not sets the scene, when we engage in a play or cinematic production we become part of it, persistently trying to figure out this cleverly written plot with our Holmes' deerstalker hats on and magnifying glass out. We take on the role of the detective, hoping and praying we are wrong, then in a flash, there it comes the inevitable twist in the tale, which often sends us reeling with the notion we knew nothing all along. We connect so deeply with the characters that if they are told a hurtful truth it is as though our own dreams have been shattered. In their joy we celebrate and in their sadness we feel sorrow yet it is all part of the journey. The reasons the film industry is so popular is due to the fact that humans as a species enjoy comedy, tragedy and drama as long as it is far enough away of course from our own life. We wish to feel scared, excited, teary eyed and much more, as long as ultimately we know it not to be real.

The heart-warming feeling and memories of watching an old classic or a childhood favourite. Isn't it odd then that we seem not to be able at times to find our own car/house keys when leaving for work, yet can recite vast amounts of complex dialogue from a treasured movie? This is due to our long and short memory faculties having completely different constructs, that is the sheer complexity of our brain. But it also has a lot to do with our focus, our attention! When engrossed in a film we take in all the information yet in our daily lives we are so used to thinking either in the past or the future we lose that much needed focus. When you do things, whatever they may be, give yourself the precious option of time, allow yourself to become the act, try to do things purposefully, be kind to yourself! They say "patience is a virtue" let that be your truest one.

Whilst compiling this chapter it has become evident that only the purest forms of creativity without an objective serve to benefit humanity indefinitely. You might respond with, "yes, but a cure for ailments is far more beneficial to humankind!" Maybe so and with all the stem cell research and preventative measures we may not have the defects and disease we have now in the future. But to try without adequate awareness to play what some may call 'God', will always bring with it irreversible consequences, we now have genetic modification, this could prevent a child forming or being born with an insufferable disease but then how far do we push that envelope? We all know the direction this is heading. Candy store babies! Blue eyes, green eyes, brown eyes, how tall we want them to be, male or female and on and on till they become an object of fashion or aesthetics. Regardless of this soothsaying, how far we push the boundaries of this reality and materialistic world will show just how significant the repercussions will be. We so often ask the question, "if we could" as opposed to asking, "if we should". There has and always will be humanistic travesties, our focus will just be redirected to a different cause, the universe has a will and a way! And to think we can control the order of things is in very similar respects, akin to King Canute trying to hold back the tides.

We now have weather modification, we treat nature as our playground, to do so as we please, safe in the comfort we may be able to right some of the wrongs. This invariably will cause humans to create more problems than before, even with the greatest will in the world and best intentions at heart, we could just as easily create a Frankenstein's monster (figuratively speaking). This is not to say we shouldn't try our best to ease the suffering of the many appalling illnesses, it is just to simply say that hindsight is a wonderful thing, and an awareness now may stop carelessness then. On the other side of the coin, maybe if we could also put the same level of effort into solving more humanitarian issues as we do with our attempts and efforts to go further, to advance, with empathy instead of greed and self-pride at the forefront the change we seek could be on the horizons or maybe what happens, happens and that's okay too. You see it's not to try to change what's already transpired, but to just reflect on it, and learn from it, to sit with it with no time frame, as only then may we get a clearer picture of what occurred and thus spread awareness, that is the key for halting future repetition. One thing is for certain the more we choose to become mindful the more the future becomes immaterial. The next big thing we may have to contend with is the developing enhancement of Artificial Intelligence, which appears incredible on the surface, but this could also be an answer to a question to which no-one ever asked! Or maybe that is just the natural progression of things! As our rapidly increasing desire to create and manufacture profusely continues this very thing may be humanity's undoing. Remember we see beauty in nature, but see aesthetics in our fabrication.

On a leaving note to this chapter ask yourself these questions…

- Why do you feel compelled at times to create something?
- Does that feeling come from deep within?
- Does that feeling feel bigger than you?
- Is this a yearning to create something new and unique?

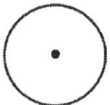

MIND/BODY

The psyche is the human mind in its entirety, formed into two parts, the conscious mind and the subconscious mind. The conscious mind is your logical mind, it receives information from your five senses, it is where you think, allowing for you to communicate with yourself, problem-solve and organise an abundance of information to form a conceivable concept. It is where you rationalise, helping you to make sense of all that is around. Logic rules the day in the conscious mind, however this side of the psyche does not dictate our physical automations, our actions are almost exclusively controlled by the subconscious mind.

This mind is largely ruled by emotions, instincts and learnt behaviour, its primary function is to help us meet our needs and urges, reproduction, sustenance, thirst, safety, intimacy and much more. It is a very powerful force and can be somewhat overbearing, it does not reason nor change, it simply acts. Often commanding your every movement, it is theorised that 90% of your brain's power is used up by the subconscious mind, yet only 10% of the brain's power is given to the conscious mind. This may have given rise to the frequently used phrase 'we only use 10% of our potential'. We can think of an action like, I want to pick up that pen and have a will to do so, instantaneously the subconscious mind will take over in the process of retrieving said item. It forms our robotic side, if it was the only mind we had we would still be very distinguishable from automatons because of the sheer wealth of emotions that reside there. It does however run on a very specific programme. Everything is subliminally registered, whether we are aware of it or not, we hear so much in our lives "practice makes perfect" and this is down to this very entity. It has a desire to win, to strive, to surpass in its every pursuit. Impulses, addictions and habits are all governed by this mind, it can help you become an incredibly talented artist or pianist but can also assist you in your rapid demise. Together these two phenomenal minds appear to work seamlessly to determine our actions, from the thought to the task, they can bring about success or loss, happiness or anxiety, accolades or frustrations. It is how we put them to use, that we prove triumphant. We are eternal creatures of habit, sometimes to our favour! Sometimes to our failure!

There can be a plethora of negative impacts to our lives that if not addressed in a timely fashion can cause a person's life to spiral out of control indefinitely. Whether you are trying to quit an addiction, find yourself in a rut or staying in a toxic relationship, it is all down to the traits encompassed by the subconscious mind. In its need to advance and perfect our techniques it creates habitual behaviours, this can be extremely advantageous but can also cause many disadvantages in the process. It has a need to acquire structure and routine in our lives. When something appears out of the ordinary it brings about feelings of dread and fear. It can cause our whole bodies to tense up as a way of protection, we all have primeval instincts. This is our innate ability to see new potentially dangerous situations in the interest of self-preservation.

This has helped humans survive perceived threats for millennia and still to this day serves us as a brilliant defence mechanism, although it can also be our unsheathed sword often causing us more harm than it serves to protect. We have to be reliant on these very instincts. What our minds perceive as a threat or a dangerous situation in our modern lives is vastly different to say a prehistoric predator. Past traumatic events we hold in our memory, stressful situations and negative environments all can and do trigger this survival instinct, causing people much distress along the way. An increase in heartbeat, over production from our adrenal glands, panic, higher energy levels, faster breathing, all culminate in a state of perpetual anxiety, and a sudden release of our stress hormone cortisol, which in fleeting spurts can help us get out of a sticky situation, but when in constant production can also cause it to act like an acid in our bodies, from which arises many bodily ailments. A strange but important aspect to this is that the subconscious mind cannot differentiate our reality from an imagined negative event and starts to put things into motion internally to protect you from this looming, self-concocted, perilous occurrence. If this becomes a persistent mind/body state we can become perpetual balls of tension and this can have dire consequences on our lives, but this does not have to be the case.

Breathing techniques as exhibited by the likes of Wim Hof can assist in bringing us back to our present reality and calm the mind, plus the famous ice therapy can also help boost our depleted immune system brought on by our anxieties and stress. Cognitive behavioural therapy and mindful meditation can serve to help relieve this curse too.

But one of the most powerful tools we have at our disposal is hypnosis. The word 'hypnosis' is derived from the Greek God Hypnos meaning 'sleep'. He was the son of Nix (the nights) and resided in a big cave in the underworld where the River Lethe (forgetfulness) flowed.

Hypnosis was given this name due to the fact that when hypnotised, a person is subliminally cast into a sleep-like state, hypnos (sleep) osis (condition). The preconception of hypnosis is that of a humorous act, with which audience members are lined up on stage, placed comfortably, yet nervously, into seats as the star of the show proceeds to cast a spell onto the unwitting participants. Then once the hypnotiser merely clicks a finger the seated members can act out a whole manner of things, turning the gleeful audience into fits of laughter. Although in recent times people are losing their prejudices towards this practice and are starting to wake up to the possibilities, therefore starting to use it in a much more rewarding way.

The non-persistent nature of hypnosis is only seen by those that attend these sessions to be of certain use, but not an outright eradicator for their many problems. Addiction therapy, with the use of hypnosis, has been around for some time, and in certain cases to great effect, but the vastness in which it can assist people in so many other aspects of their lives is mostly lost on the populous. The reason for its powerful and semi-permanent effect on our psyche is as follows, when in a sleep-like trance we exit our beta brainwave (focused state) and enter our Alpha brainwave (restful state) to a deeper state of hypnosis our Theta brainwave and finally the deepest state of hypnosis the Delta brainwave. Exactly the same as how we would, when we go from reading a book in bed, to turning the lights off, to falling asleep, and then of course deep sleep. The difference being, with sleep we enter a state of reduced consciousness, as in contrast with hypnosis this is where an artificially induced rest state in which a person has a heightened suggestibility, and where suppressed memories may also be experienced.

The fascinating trick is whilst under the so-called spell, the administrator has a direct line to our subconscious mind and its rigidly stubborn programming, whether we are counting back from a thousand or counting sheep, listening to the noises around us, thinking thoughts or paying absolutely zero attention to the therapist, the visualisation and verbal repetition in which they orate is taken in nonetheless by the subconscious. This immensely powerful side of our mind, which can at times render our willpower futile when we need it most, can also be tamed and nurtured through this practice. From our fears and irrational phobias to living a systematically mundane existence due to habitual behaviour, it can all be rewritten with time and focused effort. This part of our psyche cannot reason, it can only listen, perhaps that narrative is negative, perhaps positive, but take it in as fact, is exactly what it will do. If you get down about yourself and your situation and become self-critical, constantly bringing yourself to heel, or if you have a humdrum affinity with life or about the environment you reside or even your chosen career, your mind will take all of this information in and will continue to treat this as a persistent threat causing tension throughout your entire body, as though in anticipation of a metaphoric car crash, the result is that we are essentially causing ourselves untold mischief by continuously being in this state. Painfully tender back muscles, permanently taut neck muscles, cluster headaches, migraines, stress rashes right through to digestive issues such as Irritable Bowel Syndrome and the like. One of the most detrimental effects attributed to anxiety is the powerful way it can weaken our immune system, all that a hypnotherapist does efficiently is call through to your subconscious and with a calming repetitive voice, proceeds to tell it that everything is fine. You are handling it, no need to worry, it has already passed. This is how we change our circumstances by reciting powerfully positive affirmations.

Over a few sessions this starts to form new neurological pathways, thus alleviating the stress in a natural way. If we have an addiction or seem to be stuck in a particular pattern that is less than desirable, this process can take a fair bit longer to achieve its desirable goal.

Undeniably it can't fail to lift the curse, as although these trains of thoughts are extremely well ingrained in each of us, the making of new positive pathways will, given time replace the old ones, which will eventually fade away. It is not too dissimilar to rewriting a record on an old tape, once this has taken effect that overbearing will to act a certain way, gravitate towards hurtful actions or think certain thoughts becomes no longer prominent, and we get a chance for once in our lives to write our own record which could be our personal chart topper.

Once we let go of all that negativity and start to appreciate life with a positive mindset, all of life's hang-ups will no longer be an issue, a once bitten twice shy attitude.

We have two inherent fears, the fear of falling and the fear of loud noises, everything else is the result of past experiences and taught conceptual phobias.

Sleep

A third of our entire life is taken up by our sleep and restful periods. Each person is fully aware of just how imperative a good night's sleep is to their bodies and minds, and when on the odd occasion we build up a sleep debt through either work commitments, worry or stress it can give rise to untold mental and physical issues exhibited throughout our daily lives. From thought processing, task mastering or simply our mood, the effects of inadequate rest can take a heavy toll, not just on a personal level and the many health implications, but on those we interact with: our family, friends and even work colleagues. Lower mood stabilising hormonal production, weakened immune system and lethargy are just the tip of the iceberg, when it comes to the multifaceted afflictions that can be directly attributed to a person's lack of sleep. It can also be one of the most important considerations when it comes to how much we are able to experience life in its fullest form. So what can cause this lack of our very much needed slumber? Apart from an obvious physical ailment i.e. headaches, back aches, toothache, the four main reasons we accrue a sleep debt are, mental issues, family/relationship issues, our career and of course technology! We could put these all under one umbrella and say, our minds. Yes, it is our own mind that starts to become the thorn in our side when it comes to sleep deprivation. We start to play out scenarios in our head as soon as that light goes out if we are ill at ease, something simple like a lecture we have to give at work the very next day, trying to reason an annoyance we have, say a car constantly parked over our driveway for instance by an ignorant neighbour or dreaming up how we would like our lives to turnout. So what is the culprit here? you may have worked that one out. It's pretty obvious isn't it? Our malevolent friend the ego! It seems to whisper sweet nothings into our ears, causing us to feel distress and doubtful about the situation, "Are you sure you are up to the task tomorrow? Is everything you typed up to scratch? What if you lose your voice? What if you say the wrong thing and they poke fun at you?" and so anxiety ensues. Or it starts to pick up on the petulant neighbour scene! It may say, "who do they think they are, treating you with such disregard? They're practically saying you are not important and they will do whatever they like, you can't let them get away with it. This calls for action!

"Show them you are not one to be messed around with!" and on and on, until your blood starts to boil over and that vital shut eye becomes the last thing on your mind. It causes a false confidence which can, if not reasoned with, initiate a rapid escalation and altercation to occur. It gets you to believe you are the only one that matters, you are the most important.

Although a credible annoyance and a slight inconvenience, we do not know what stresses or even traumatic events our neighbours are dealing with, it may have only been for a day or so and only a slight overhang making it a bit tricky to navigate our car through into the driveway. The neighbour may not be feeling 100%, they could have lost their job, have an illness in their family or even a tragedy. Unless we reason with people with an open heart how can we help to heal? Okay, you could say, "no this neighbour has been doing it for weeks and we tried telling them but they said it's a free country and they just don't care!" This is a harder situation in which to remain calm of course, but let's try to understand and reason this out anyway, ask yourself what entity is controlling their actions? Now do you see! And so, empathy has to be shown. This will have an alleviating effect and a clearer mind in which you can approach and handle the situation better. If you don't, that whisper will get louder and the call for revenge could be your next strategy, a 'two wrongs don't make a right!' if you will.

When we reason and try to be mindful of the situations in our lives we rationalise and process them in a noticeably more positive light, often giving us the answer to the problem we sorely seek. If you quieten or even silence the inferior voice and learn to show compassion and understanding with the confidence and contentment in who you are, all that chatter will vanish and the much needed sleep that had been escaping you will sweep over like a warm blanket.

Further ways we can assist ourselves in obtaining a restful night's sleep are, as we have mentioned technology, namely blue light sources, abstaining from devices such as smartphones, laptops and tablets will help in resetting our natural circadian rhythm, the natural process of night and day has been ingrained in humans through the history of our evolution. To sync back up with nature on the sunrise/sunset periods will help get you back to yourself in a matter of weeks. A preferable option (if you struggle to switch off at night) is to start reading a physical book as this will take your mind off the daily stresses allowing for a seamless transition into the land of nod. When at times we go through episodes of insomnia, a week's break away from all modern living, and a reconnection with nature will have a profound effect on the psyche. Easier said than done but hugely beneficial, nonetheless. What about night workers? In today's culture of consumerism and global conglomerates' need for greed we have fallen into an irreversible trap of using all the time we have in which to capitalise on profits, so the period we have set aside and evolved with for rest since early humans existence is now seen as fair game. Although massively unfavourable to an individual to have to work through the difficult nightshift, unemployment, security and debt forcibly compels a person to take those opportunities whenever they arise, however undesirable they seem.

We are an extremely adaptable species! But to go against 200,000 years or possibly millions of years of evolution as diurnal active beings is no mean feat. There are certain ways to help in this matter though, as we know it is night's darkness that assists our sleep pattern, the reason why? The pineal gland (given the name for its structure's similarities in shape to that of a pine cone) or as Rene Descartes once called it, 'the principle seat to the soul' also referred to as the third eye, but we will get to that later. Its predominant role is to halt production of serotonin and increase the production of melatonin, a derivative of serotonin, which in turn is formed from its precursor tryptophan, an amino acid we obtain through our diets via protein based foods. Have you ever wondered why on Christmas Day or Thanksgiving not long after we have devoured the delicious turkey dinner and began to watch our favourite film, with the fire roaring, that all of the family start to show signs of narcosis? That is because they have a belly full of the best foods, lots of carbs, pigs in blankets and plenty of turkey all washed down with a favourite tipple or two. Turkey is one of the most abundant sources of tryptophan, but any overindulgence of carbs and high intake of proteins will have this same effect, a nut roast will do the job just as well, combined with the warmth, happy times and no more stresses of buying and wrapping presents, all go together to create a perfect environment for a winters siesta.

Now getting back to the pineal gland, as you are aware its primary function is to start the production of melatonin, which in turn has many uses in the central nervous system, most importantly it helps regulate our sleep patterns. Melatonin production is stimulated by darkness and inhibited by light. Once the retina detects a light source on its many light sensitive nerve cells it sends a signal to the suprachiasmatic nucleus (SCN) synchronising the SCN to the day night cycle. Nerve fibres relay this information from the SCN to paraventricular nuclei (PVN) then through the spinal cord and onto the superior cervical ganglia, and from there it finally reaches the pineal gland where melatonin can either be produced or halted. So, as we can be sure by now you are fully aware of the impact light emitting electronic devices has on the amount of time it can take to finally drift off and get that much needed rest in order for you to wake up the next day feeling refreshed and in a positive mood, ready for whatever experiences await you.

Dreams and their functions

At night when our heads hit that soft, cool pillow and our eyelids meet in the middle, we go through different stages of sleep. The first stage, REM, happens once we are asleep and our conscious mind is switched off. In essence our subconscious mind is still very much operational and this can bring about our dream states.

It is thought that we dream in intervals of between five and twenty minutes at a time, and we can have up to six dreams a night, whether we can recollect them in the morning or not. So why do we dream? There is much speculation to this. It could be a way of processing information collected throughout our day, a way of self-analysing. Dreams could be images we display to our unconscious part of the brain or a way in which we represent subconscious wishes and desires we hold for ourselves in the future. Other accepted ideas are that it helps people develop our cognitive capabilities, prepares them for possible future threats and a state in which they can bring together contradictory or overwhelmingly highly complex notions as to save them from the unsettling feelings they would cast upon themselves if they were consciously aware of such thoughts.

Dreams tend to be full of vivid experiences and sensations, hence the reason why we cannot disassociate ourselves from knowing that it isn't reality and that we are asleep. Often, the ideas racing around our minds before we drift off form the dream experience. Repressed emotions also seem to play a major part too. Dreams can be like flashbacks to memories with wonderfully melancholic undertones, the sounds of the ice cream truck that use to frequent our street, the tastes, the aromas all play into this feeling of nostalgia. But just as they have pleasurable notes there has to be painful flashbacks too, a particular forgotten memory of a loved one we have lost, they can leave a distasteful flavour in our mouth. They can conjure up hardships we have fought with and in other cases they may bring back a certain ill feeling, possibly how we used to feel as a child in unbearable circumstances, witnessing terrible arguments, and so we start to envelop these sensations, once again becoming that frightened child which can invoke a powerful myriad of emotions. So, to summarise, dreams help us compute massive amounts of data and process this information in a way that it is possible for us to understand subconsciously and in turn utilised to benefit our very being.

Interpretations of dreams and their relevance and many hidden meanings

Whether you have dreamt that your teeth are falling out or you are running backwards in an attempt to evade capture by the talons of a monster, there seems to always be an interpretation to each of them, in which we may learn something about ourselves from the complex settings. We will try to go through three hypothesised groups, relationships, sexual concepts and feelings of embarrassment. If we are in danger, falling or being chased this could mean we have interpersonal conflicts in our lives (relationships). If there are experiences of flying, sexual encounters, finding money or eating sumptuous and exotic food this could help towards formulating our own sexual concepts.

Lastly, have you ever found that halfway through a dream you are suddenly naked or inappropriately dressed, failing an exam, arriving late to an occasion or losing teeth. These type of dreams could be associated with fear of embarrassments and or social concerns. The list is endless to exactly what we dream of and the meanings behind them. But it seems to be widely accepted that it is a process which serves to help us develop cognitively and emotionally, which in turn helps each of us make sense of our lives and our environments, therefore of huge relevance.

It would be an agreeable thought to have, that whilst asleep all we did was dream, but the downside to sleep is the night terrors that inevitably pop up on the odd occasion or in some cases for periods of weeks at a time, like everything we have to see the good and the bad to experience it as a whole. So what do nightmares teach us and why do we have them?

Some of the main reasons we have nightmares is down to our mental state. If we are anxious, have forms of depression, or suffer with PTSD, we can have recurring episodes of night terrors, constantly replaying a traumatic event. Night terrors mainly affect children from between the ages of three to six, and most grow out of this phase. It can also be hereditary, they seem to occur in the earliest part of sleep, and last several minutes, but can happen multiple times on any given night. Their impact on a child's mental health isn't deemed to be long lasting therefore, it is widely accepted that they cause no serious psychological harm to the child. The only real impact it can have is they seem to wake from a deep sleep due to excitement or anxiety brought on by the terror, can wake more easily from a sudden noise or having to empty their bladder.

These episodes can be triggered through different factors, namely tiredness, a fever or medication. The best thing as adults is to let the nightmare play out, although this can be hard to do, as to bear witness to such conceived traumas as loving adults we often feel compelled to intervene, but this will cause more anguish to the child upon trying to wake them. In the confusion they may not recognise you and start to feel more agitated if you try to comfort them, it is a process that we can minimise by taking heed of the triggers, but it is something that ultimately has to run its course. You should try not to get too emotionally involved however hard that might be and see it as a process, as opposed to the hurt you think your child is encountering. The child will on most occasions not even remember anything come the next morning, or even be conscious of it throughout the day.

So why do adults have nightmares? As we have said, how you feel in your life and what your mental state is in will have an impact on your sleep and subsequent nightmares. It may unconsciously try to get you to live up to your fears, rationalise the problems you have mentally stored, get you to see the importance of such things you have disregarded, or traumatic events you have buried deep inside you. As distressing as it may feel, the positives to take are that they can help you accept certain things and really understand them which will result in you being able to come to terms with them on a deep emotional level. Another benefit is they can also allow you to get to the root of an internal turmoil, alleviating deeply depressed thoughts thus bringing them to the surface for you to deal with in a more constructive way.

The extra little things we can do to assist in how much quality sleep we obtain is to eat high sources of tryptophan. Yes you can acquire melatonin via pill form in certain countries but the doses may be too high or too low for any individual and because it comes in pure form it is harder for the body to adequately regulate. A much better solution is to ingest natural occurring sources, that way your body can utilise and make the amount it needs. Highly potent nutritional sources for melatonin production are dairy products and meat proteins or alternative protein sources for the vegan and vegetarian diet, legumes and nuts, the most abundant source coming from pistachios. Another high source is fresh fruit, particularly berries. A small glass of tart sour cherry juice before bed can be just the ticket for getting that much anticipated shut eye. Also grains and seeds, too. You can start to see why a balanced diet is absolutely paramount to a healthy body and mind.

Nutrition and a balanced diet

Most people try to become healthy through their diet in order for their body to be as fit and healthy as it can be, coupled with physical activity. But rarely do we consider how a healthy diet can also benefit us in a mental capacity. To exercise and eat well will undeniably have a vastly positive effect on our bodies, allowing for us to fight infections and disease and be more able bodied, and so not having as many life-long ailments which might in turn permit us to be on this planet just that little bit longer.

The most powerful effect though lies in how it also assists our mental health through the natural process. To have a lean and fit body will of course have an uplifting effect on our daily lives through the confidence it may bestow upon us. But what is transparent is just how much of an amazing impact it has on our minds and mental clarity!

Being present, problem-solving, our moods and all round passion for life. It goes some way to help in our avoidance of mental issues such as depression and anxiety. If at times we develop these torrid issues we generally don't feel good and lock ourselves away, which can lead to more serious issues. When this vicious cycle is formed, we are told to "go and see a doctor" and so we do. There, we are assessed, given a diagnosis and prescribed numerous mood lifting drugs, which can have a great effect but because we are all individuals and what is thought to be appropriate on a wide spectrum may not necessarily be the correct amount we require. This can invariably cause a yoyo effect.

Trials and tests help to give pharmaceutical companies a statistic from the data but not an accurate enough figure for an individual person. The premise from the GP and the pharmaceutical world is that in time you will see the same benefit. They work, there is no doubt about it, but the length of time it can take and the negative side effects can take their toll. This cascading effect, in which the intake of such substances leads to more negative actions on other parts of our body and mind, unless they take an individual test for each patient they cannot account for the impacts, or to what level the person will benefit from them.

Our emotions are governed by the dominating part of the mind and only felt by our inferior mind and because every person has slightly differing unique structures and defects the actual levels of chemical and hormonal release can be significant. When the subconscious starts to interpret and control outside and inside factors, it initiates the release of certain substances as a way of allowing the conscious mind to become aware and feel the pending emotion. But the problem for a certain amount of people is the inability to control or produce the required amount due to shortcomings in their brain and so the release maybe ineffective and could have dire consequences. Our next objective is to try to gain help through various specialists, cognitive behavioural therapy and psychiatry therapy, which can change our understanding of the problem, allowing for it to be accepted and dealt with appropriately.

But let's say that there wasn't a defect in our output but that the problem stemmed solely from the amount of chemicals that were made available to our body via the intake of these vital substances in our diets. This can be detrimental to our outlook. A much more vigilant approach is to consider what sustenance we consume and make available subsequently providing a natural cure to our bodies and mind. (This is only effective in mild cases but will still help enormously even in the more extremely cases in parallel with other forms of assistance.) In this way we give ourselves a chance to change the course without any of the negative side effects. This is an approach we should take regardless, if we have any major issues with our libido. Our lust for life could be left waiting due to the simple fact that we just cannot seem to put our finger on the issue. Then say we receive bad news and fall further into that pit of depression, whereas if we start to become mindful of just what we eat, we can help in all processes of the mind/body experience in a homeostasis way, not in a vital temperature control/ water regulatory sense, but in a harmonious sense relating to the dynamic state of equilibrium between the mind and body, providing ourselves with optimal functionality. You must remember this is not to say we should not take the advice of specialists or not take the drugs they offer, rather that we should also incorporate natural resources to enhance the effectiveness.

Lymphatic system

Just to touch on this often neglected but vitally important system we all harbour within our bodies. You might have only reflected upon it if you or your family have been stricken with a form of lymphoma. Or you may be aware of the many nodes that link this system. One of its main functions is to balance the water content of the blood and filter its plasma, its most importance contribution is to create the many T cells that fight infection and stop cancers forming. Small muscle contractions allow it to push the lymphatic fluid up to drains in the chest and neck areas, exercise and the like all assist this process, there are a few things we can do to help further, an obvious one being to drink plenty of water to flush this complex structure, also very gentle massaging in the correct regions will all contribute to a free flowing efficient and functional lymphatic system.

Emotions

Emotions are an instrument we use to experience life, to participate and feel the very thing we call existence. They are expressions to convey who we are and how we feel which can leave an impression on another person, they can help protect us, to gain an understanding and give ourselves entirely to this journey. They are also the very essence of what makes our reality feel real. We even appear real in a sense when we display our emotions, how could we exist without them? Would we simply become awesome automatons? Possibly! To simplify exactly just what emotions are and how they are conveyed let's look at our power over them or more importantly the power they have over us.

Let's try to simplify this process in our minds, take a small vial for instance, into which we might add a variety of chemicals (hormonal substances), now we will leave just what and how much up to the subconscious mind. Say we are in a troubling or sticky situation or perhaps we meet someone for the first time and take an instant dislike to said person. We may then try to reason as to why we do not care so much for them using the quote 'never judge a book by the cover'. What is going on in the subconscious mind is that it will return to past experiences and make a judgement call. How the person appears, how the person portrays themselves, are they loud and confident? Are they quiet with a subtle smile and glint in their eyes? All of this information gets translated by your subconscious side, it will either allow you to feel a perceived future threat brought on by past experiences with similar personalities and traits or it will force you to close up and cause a social distancing to occur all via the amount of chemical hormonal substances it releases into our imagined vial. Which is then felt by the conscious mind and actioned by the body.

Happiness, sadness, anger, surprise, fear, disgust, were thought to be the six emotions humans exhibited but it is considerably more. From confusion to satisfaction there could be as many as twenty seven felt by a person. They are all unique concoctions from a distinct mixture of chemicals, and when mixed in just the right way they bring about the multitude of sensations you feel daily. This is why it can be so difficult to kick a drug habit.

Ecstasy being given the name as a result of the intensely euphoric feeling cast over a person who has consumed it. This is because is triggers a chain reaction inside them which offers a wealth of feel- good chemicals that overwhelm and take over their consciousness. But that lustful infatuation can cause severe harm too! as it is the ultimate escapism and the degrees of intensity have to be increased to attain the same experience.

Then we have heroin and now fentanyl which is causing so many lost souls to lose everything in one fell swoop. It's the same premise but to a much lesser extent why we crave attention and popularity. It is that sudden release of dopamine amongst others that makes us feel so happy and in constant need for more. However, Dopamine is also a neurotransmitter which helps the body function and is present throughout our bodies at all times. It is signalled by the reward system which can also offer up many benefits. Having said that, there are substantially more favourable feel good chemicals to the body and mind when increased in the system, they are released at times of love, connection, compassion and vigour. Oxytocin, endorphins and serotonin in higher doses are released when we feel content and happy.

Oxytocin is a hormone released by the pituitary gland - also referred to as the cuddle hormone or love hormone because it is released when we bond socially or hug people close to us. Endorphins can act on opiate receptors in the brain, they contribute to reducing pain and boosting pleasure which could then lead to an all-round feeling of well-being. They are released in response to pain or stress but can also be released whilst partaking in certain activities, eating pleasurable foods, whilst exercising and in the act of sex. It is also released by the pea sized pituitary gland.

Serotonin is predominantly produced in the intestines (although to a lesser extent formed in the brain and central nervous system) and is the result of the breakdown of amino acids namely tryptophan. This neurotransmitter is stored in the blood and used by the central nervous system for many functions, the positive boost it can give to the mind is a massive benefit, hence if we do not make enough available to our body via our diet the consequences can become extremely obvious.

It affects our mood, digestion, sexual appetite, and numerous other bodily functions. It can be over produced whilst exercising and can give that 'top of the world' feeling and a vital second wind. There are also hormones that can make us feel sad too, but it is the hormonal imbalances that lead to depression and anxiety.

Emotional traits

We might see a particular person and have them pinned down to a certain emotional characteristic. The grumpy old man stereotype, the mild and meek woman, the happy go lucky shopkeeper, the stern librarian, the shy timid child or even the hot-headed angry so and so. Once we repetitively see a character in our lives display biased emotions we begin to categorise them by that very thing, with thoughts of, 'isn't Debbie always bubbly, happy and always up for a laugh?' or 'poor John he always looks down in the dumps'. True as it may seem, this forms the way we perceive the many people who often cross our path, and how we create personalities for our family, friends and acquaintances. Also, how you are perceived by others will be completely different in every case.

Going back to our emotional mind and its impact on an individual with a defect or impairment in the amount of hormonal substances their bodies may produce can result in that person being unable to show the variety of emotions that you might be able to display.

Another way of thinking about it is, as hard as it is to disassociate a person from the emotions they show and act upon. They do not have ultimate control, they can only try to influence their actions or learn to become more aware and mindful as a way of calming the effect. But what if it is ingrained into their mind from time immemorial? Then the powerful subconscious mind is in the driving seat. So, instead of outcasting people for showing negative emotions we should sympathise and help them see things in a different or more positive light. We cannot cast the first stone. We too show many emotions on any given day at any given time - some of the basics are excitement, contempt, joy, sadness, fear, disgust, surprise, anger and happiness. Each one an important response, but as with anything, too many negative responses can call for a rethink.

Visual and audible experiences can also alter our mood and output to the world, they can have a huge impact on how we feel within their surroundings. Emotions are just a tool which we utilise to feel alive in this reality, with every fibre of our body. Our very existence would be so much less and diminished without them, as we could not appreciate all that is if it weren't for their qualities, but they are far from who we are.

It is natural to show emotions, we shouldn't hope to suppress them, telling someone to buckle up or it doesn't really matter or stopping a child from expressing themselves will only lead to internal anguish and neurosis. Imagined or emotional pain can be felt in exactly the same way as physical pain. This is why it is crucial to stay detached from the pain, feel it but never identify with it. You may have seen in a history lesson the images of the Vietnamese Mahayana Buddhist monk Thich Quang Duc who set himself aflame (Self-immolation) in protest towards the Vietnam regime at a busy Saigon road intersection, an unbelievably powerful scene. We have the preconception that the monk must have been able to exhibit extreme self-discipline therefore, master his own mind in such a way as to not feel the pain by blocking it out completely! The truth is he would have probably felt the pain at a much higher intensity than most people, yet the key to his secret lay in the way he was able to disassociate himself from the pain, therefore realise it was a sensation of the body /mind experience and not an actuality. This is something we can all incorporate (to a lesser degree! of course) when we at times encounter emotional trauma. We can also have our emotions played with and exploited by the people we interact with on a daily basis. Emotions can cause us to lose our cool, lose our heads, and ultimately lose ourselves, Winston Churchill once stated "You cannot reason with a tiger once your head is in its mouth" for once the emotion has gotten a hold of you and is felt, it is extremely difficult to back away and contain or refrain from the action it can force you to display. If only we try to understand and become mindful of these emotions, then we can learn to judge them for what they are and not for what act they might compel us to do. Feel them erupt but never concede to them. We are of course discussing the less desirable sides to our emotions as the more beautiful aspects are to be cherished and engaged with in their entirety always.

Brain structural defects

We have discussed how abnormalities in the brain's structure can cause noticeable changes to a person's mental wellbeing however what happens to a person who has damage to a large region of the brain? What are some of the prolific consequences for that person and how might they be perceived by society as a result? Someone with damage to the prefrontal cortex through an accident or stunted formation in the womb will have tendencies to perform tasks in a poor manner. Also, their inhibitions to impulses can be impaired, they might even experience blunted emotional responses too. Someone who has committed a heinous crime may have abnormalities in this region of the brain also, reduced connections between the vmPFL which is responsible for such sentiments as empathy and guilt and the amygdala which mediates fear and anxiety. This can nullify the person from attaching these specific emotions to their actions and to their victims, another poignant area is the frontal lobe! An injury to this part may prevent people from making good decisions. Also acts of love can be the same as an addict's response, the emotional control and need to be strong become overwhelmed. It can also increase irritability within the individual, which could alter their mood and result in an inability to regulate behavioural proficiency. So, what can this mean when we bear witness to such horrific crimes? Our instant response is to persecute and make assumptions. This is not to say we should sympathise with the persons of interest, but become aware of all the factors that surround the circumstances.

Once the crime has been committed we throw the book at them, rightly or wrongly, apart from our final judgement of 'is this person of mental soundness or is this person mentally disabled?' A fair judgement, but let's revise our understandings at this point.

We have established the subconscious mind controls 90% of the brain's power, it has inherited beliefs and prejudices etched into it from our earliest days, it dictates our emotions which in turn serves to dictate ourselves, we can have the wrong or insufficient chemicals in our bodies, whether that be from our diets or defects in our genetic make-up which could allow for an important hormonal imbalance to occur and lastly we have an overwhelming ego! We can feel no love or sympathy for anyone after the act has been committed. But what we can do is reason with them, and more importantly become aware earlier on socially and governmentally. If we start to appreciate the magnitude of impacts this can have and understand each factoring contribution, we may be able to cut the head off the snake so to speak. In childhood, adolescents and even in young adults it might be possible to make a significant change not with the will of the world, but with a mindful approach, allowing for an ease of passage in healing the unfortunate. Abuse creates abuse! Hate breeds hate and love conquers all. Love, compassion and empathy are the three keys to the universe!

Try to think of something you do consciously that isn't born out of the subconscious/emotional mind or for an emotional response, isn't instinctive or because of an influential factor or to serve the greater good. When you can answer this set of questions firmly and without doubt! only then will you understand the level of actual control you ultimately have on the actions you take.

Our dark side

We all have a dark side. As at times we all have thoughts we'd rather not think, this could be vengeance, wishing bad karma or even harm onto someone you dislike. The difference is we have the mental capacity to inhibit such thoughts, so never act upon them. If we never had that ability how restrained would we be? Our dark side maybe needed in order for us to regulate our moral compass, maybe so that we can learn to walk a mile in another person's shoes, gaining a greater understanding for why things came to light.

Memory

Memory is divided into two parts: we have implicit memory in which we collect and store data from throughout our lives and use it subconsciously to become more efficient at performing tasks. It also influences our thoughts and behaviour. The other side is explicit memory, a conscious intentional recollection of factual data, past experiences and concepts. Each memory can be broken down into three parts, encoding, storage and retrieval.

Most of our memories are stored in the subconscious, how we performed tasks and ways in which we improved, all amalgamate so that we end up in a state where we no longer have to be consciously aware of what we are doing for us to perform the actions. Whether we become aware of it or not has no relevance, in fact often when we do at times overthink an action we have enacted a thousand times we lose the flow and can perform poorly, riding a bike, brushing our teeth, tying our shoelaces or when driving a car. Although we make a conscious effort to initiate these specific jobs the subconscious mind takes over extremely quickly and with its memory and learnt behaviour it goes about its business post-haste.

The downside to this storage faculty, is that we can on occasions after experiencing something traumatic, bury the memory deep inside. This is what we call 'suppressed memories' and they can have an extreme effect on our mental state. The only way of alleviating this is to bring it back to the surface with cognitive behavioural therapy, hypnotherapy or psychotherapy. If we don't deal with these suppressions we could hamper our chances of living a well-rounded life! As John Lennon once quoted, 'there are two basic motivating forces, fear and love'. When we are afraid, we pull back from life, when we are in a state of love we open up to all that life has to offer with passion, excitement and acceptance. The point being we may all have these suppressed emotions and memories whether we recollect why or not.

If you feel you have a mental blockage regarding certain aspects of significance In your life, then to go into yourself and find the answer could in itself be the cure, even simple things that are of no danger can still impede your experience. So our memory helps our minds make appropriate choices, keeps us from encountering somewhat unfavourable situations and helps us perform to the best of our physical abilities. We can't talk about memory without mentioning the cases in which there becomes an impermanent or degenerative disease of the brain and its dire consequences. With age comes a slow decline in the recollective part of our memory. We can use subtle but effective tools to keep it as fresh as possible, mental exercises and the like.

What about the more progressive and detrimental failings such as Mixed Dementia or Alzheimer's? In these devastatingly tragic cases whether it be a friend or close relative we see before our very eyes the person we have known intimately for many years start to lose elements of their character, it can be a crude and systematic dismantling of the 'I', from the tiniest of traits, to how they interact with you on a personal level, then as it takes a real hold they can forget who we are completely.

It is truly heart-breaking to see someone you have admired for so long fall victim to this horrible illness and lose who they are in the process, their persona, their character, their identity. We start to think of how we used to envisage them, from their strict ways, their sense of humour to the affection they have shown towards us, this once strong minded, independent figure can soon become fragile and helpless which ultimately crushes all who witness. Even after this family member or friend has lost the ability to remember the smallest of things and is unable to recollect who we are any longer with a gaze that used to be felt as recognition, there is an awareness in ourselves that even though they are lost to us in a mental capacity, the soul, the spirit, the very essence of that person is still very much present and so we can at least take comfort from that and treasure it for eternity.

Sometimes we can even get nostalgic about the historical past and how life was. It may not have played any direct role in our life yet we long for the past and its sepia tonal colours and atmospheric settings as they seem to instil in us a strong sentiment that we belong, yet we can become fearful of an imagined future! This is strange but true. The past and future are conceived and activated by the same parts of the brain, and it seems many of us choose to spend the majority of time dwelling in these specific domains. It would be wise to enter, find a comfy chair for a brief moment, contemplation but then exit and return to the present, for what you think you are gaining reliving or predicting past and future occurrences you are losing in your now.

Mind control

How powerful is the mind? Not only can it cause tremendous amounts of pain and suffering it can also heal almost anything that resides within you, physiological or psychological. It can also turn into the enemy as we become the unwitting foe. How can our minds be used against us? Well we know the ego is a shrewd, self-serving character who consistently causes a person to become paranoid and instils self-doubt, but there are many other impish forms we interact with that can also use psychological warfare to our disadvantage, notably the many bullies we can come across in life. These unprincipled trolls will have undoubtably tried this unethical act and succeeded to gain that advantage. This doesn't have to be the typical playground bully taking our lunch money type. Many we see as loved ones or friends can play tricks, as a way of swaying you, not in a malicious way but maybe to protect you or for you to conform to their ways of thinking. When pure of heart it is easy to be manipulate. Naive and gullible people can be preyed upon by those they trust most. We've all seen mind tricks being performed maybe you can recollect a card trick or a guided answer. The goal is to make the person more suggestible and compliant.

Distractions, subliminal messaging all conspire towards a person being led down the garden path. It is only when we return, gauge our bearings and start to become mindful again that the mystery of the magic disappears, which can be a very useful thought to remember when trying to go down your own path and the choices you make as to not want to be forcibly led by others!

We are all now familiar with the media and governmental propaganda issues which target our beliefs and the self-negative narrative we create. But the way in which the marketing for global conglomerates use the collective conscious and ego against populations can be deemed wholly unfair at times. If a cause is worthy then to have it within arm's reach through the greater public platforms is principally and morally just. But to avidly target a human's emotions and insecurities, and so wave it under a person's nose for profit, can be viewed as dangerously unjust and unwarranted. Yet this has been the case since advertisements came into creation and is their fundamental principle. 'Sell to the classes and the masses', the problem being, it seems, that with evermore advancements in computer science, algorithms and A.I. we may fall further victim to desires we never anticipated. We are having our subconscious minds whisper to without our conscious mind being made aware, as that is where compulsions are harboured and started. Marketing algorithms see the masses of data and systematically formulate and target the vulnerable or let's say suggestable groups, which in turn causes trends and the latest fashions. Not wanting to look foolish or outcast from popularity, the ego forcefully compels people to buy into these dreams that have a chance of making them accepted even for a brief moment. But that would be akin to chasing that pot of gold at the end of the rainbow, it is fictitious, you know deep down the answer to this.

The human mind is one of the most powerful weapons at our disposal, it can hurt us and it can also heal us, it can cause strange phenomena such as people becoming maths and linguistics experts or even a fluent pianist with no formal training after a head trauma injury. It has the ability to remove restrictions put in place to protect us for example, confusing a child who has hurt themselves after falling from their bike thus distracting them from the pain. If we change their awareness and focus of the pain, the pain can be instantly lessened as a result. It can help us perform feats of superhuman strength on rare occasions, an image often springs to mind of someone lifting extremely heavy objects to save a loved one who has become trapped. It can be our best friend or our biggest enemy depending on how we treat it. Love, compassion and empathy for ourselves as well as others is a sure-fire way to gain its trust, giving it adequate rest essentially nurturing our soul will all cause a big shift in our psyche in favour of a much more vibrant and positive attitude, it can also be the most delicately fragile part of our very being.

Sigmund Freud and Carl Jung, two incredible psychoanalysts, although highly regarded and of undeniable intellect with substance and meaning, their bodies of work could still be assessed as personal opinionated matter. Freud gave us the term a 'Freudian slip' referring to the subconscious thoughts we sometimes mistakenly utter aloud, and then of course we have Jung and his amazingly insightful mind. He was also a close colleague of Freud for some years and even though he agreed with certain theorised premises of Freud's work he often discredited much too, which for better or worse was instigated by his own self-importance. They have both left us, nonetheless, an incredible understanding of the workings of the human psyche. So what led to the rapid expansion of the frontal lobe in humans which is responsible for our cognitive skills, emotional expression, memory, judgement, language, problem-solving, the ultimate command centre, which massively assisted humans with their speedy evolution and which in turn gave birth to civilisation? There are multiple theories as to why the most recently developed part of the brain was able to evolve at a unprecedented rate. All have some truth behind them, but an interesting theory is that psychedelics caused an expansion in the human consciousness through certain mind-altering natural substances. It is all speculation but an intriguing path to venture down.

What is your own concept of how much control you have over your life? It might be an honest assumption to say in percentage terms possibly between 60% and 70% as you believe if you want to do something or achieve a merit most of the time it will come to fruition! right? But when you really think about it, even the things we want are taught choices, and so are a way to please others or how we may then be perceived by others. We have inherited beliefs and concepts, coupled with factors of our lives that are out of our hands - the environment, our genetics, other people and their decisions. So how much control do we really have? It would be foolish to say we cannot have much control or say on our lives as there are an abundance of things we can do to alter this and lead an existence more befitting in order gain the most experience and enjoyment out of our life. Turning to our intuitive side would be a great start.

How do you see yourself? Maybe some of the layers are starting to fall away slightly, maybe there is some cognitive dissonance. What do you see when you look in the mirror? A mere well-wisher you say "hello" to at the start and end of each day? Are you able to distinguish your mental self from the façade? Have you ever looked in the mirror and intently gazed into the windows of the soul and after so long when the rest of the face becomes but a blur start to get a subtle sensation you are falling, a sense you are detaching from the body then arrive at the conclusion this is just a physical form we reside in, in order to bring about this reality, your character, your mind, your appearance? Whether you reflect upon yourself as beautiful, tall, short, skinny, whatever widely accepted advantage or disadvantage, it is all just a fortunate occurrence which allows you to be in existence. The real you, the true you is much deeper within, and all the meaningful answers you seek throughout your life are there to behold at all times, all it takes is mindful awareness and a connection to be made!

When we have no barriers forced upon us and no preconceptions, when we just are and trust in what will be in the same way we trust our bodies to breathe for us, our hearts to beat, our immune system to fight off infection, only then when the metaphoric shackles have been removed do we really get to live in the moment and be true to ourselves. The strangest of concepts is in science, throughout the years of research we are still not categorically certain where the actual mind resides within our bodies, only subtle hints, maybe it resides in many parts and not just the brain.

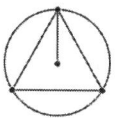

LIFE IS A PARADOX

You could say that life is a paradox as it seems to have no rational meaning! Yet we can find our own meaning throughout the journey, it can be both morbid yet also beautiful, filled with hate and also love, it has hardships and periods of serenity, we can experience heartbreak and the most special of occasions, the ups and downs, peaks and troughs of life. Isn't that the best description we can give? That existence is merely a wave with which we travel upon, trying hard to steer the course, when really we should learn to use its power, for we may fall off. Life is energy, as we are energy.

We have talked about its many quoted meanings but now it may be wise to ask yourself, what gives your life meaning or what is your purpose? Is it even necessary to have one?

Now try and truly think about your beliefs about the afterlife. Is it a recollection to something ascribed by others, or a conclusion/opinion of your own volition? Remind yourself of the analogy we have recently attributed to life, that of its similarities to a wave. Many have theorised universal energy is eternal and as electrical beings both physically and spiritually we must therefore also be eternal. We can all get mental hang ups regarding this notion 'everything has a beginning and an end' thus becoming so fixated on this idea that we take it as the undeniable truth, when in the same breath energy is eternal, has no end only change. Waves do not just have a single crest and peak they are followed by repetition like the ripples of a lake. We call it a circle of life not a straight line, we confine life into a box of rigid structure, but neglect far more reasonable premises and that might possibly be okay, but to confine our spirits by the same principles would be a travesty of great measure.

Our bodies are filled with huge amounts of tension from the daily grind and anxieties of life forever gripped in this state of a constant crushing worry, always anticipating an imminent accident, eternally bracing for impact, a heightened sense of danger for we may lose control or that things might not go according to our plan. From the way we contort our faces and the unnatural ways we find our backs and necks positioned. It could be late at night when the stresses of the day have been left behind and the pressures have been somewhat lifted, this is when we start to become aware of our bodies and once we become aware, we soon realise that we are all but a tightly wound ball of string.

From the strain in our eyes, the gripping tension in our faces with slightly clenched jaws, to the stiffness in our necks and the throbbing pressure in our temples, of course our next instinct is to try to relax, so we lower the muscles in our foreheads, drop the shoulders, run a nice hot bath or shower and possibly pour a tipple of our favourite beverage to serve as a nightcap. Then after all that we climb into our wondrously soft bed, and lie upon our sumptuously cloud-like mattress and sink our heads into the light marshmallows we call pillows. A strange sensation rushes over us, that being a feeling of tranquillity!

This gratifying relaxation being the polar opposite to how we feel for the most parts of the day, should we not feel more like this during our daily routine? Why are we so uptight? This all comes back to control, thinking we can influence every eventuality, is it natural to feel like this every single working day? Is this even sustainable? has something got to give before we address these issues? Do we surrender to the idea that it is simply part of the process! Maybe it is with just a few hang ups to consider. And possibly your career is rewarding and something you have worked extremely hard towards and so in this case you relish going back to work warts and all.

I'm sure you will have heard this saying, 'get a job you love and you'll never work a day in your life'. So maybe the trick really is to not sweat the small stuff. On the other hand maybe this isn't you and the job is just that, a job, an absolute necessity, with a partner and family to provide for, cash commitments, debt, a mortgage, a whole manner of contributing factors. It becomes pretty obvious that we should follow our dreams in order to lead a healthier balanced life, to eradicate the normality of our anxieties and stresses, but that's easier said than done.

As humans we are great procrastinators but what we excel at more so is efficiently and systematically compiling mental lists of problems. We are set up in this way to see the threat, pre-empt the worst case scenario, find faults, this is our very own internal safety protection feature of the mind and we become proficient at this. It is greatly adapted to every decision we make. We spend far more time finding problems than we do solutions, it can be as simple as an ingrained idea that education stops as soon as our schooling is over, to start a new course when we are in our mid-twenties, mid-thirties or even forty and above is preposterous. But analyse this notion, you are at a point in your life where you have gained vast amounts of experience, Check! you are in tune with who you are, Check! and are fully aware of the plethora of talents that have presented themselves to you, Check!

It begs the question, are you fully aware of the life you wish to lead as a school leaver? A college/university leaver? What you believed to be your purpose or calling most of the time was a collage of the influences around you, a wave of constant pressure and a bombardment of opinionated ideas. The only thing that was missing was a clear direction for you to head for, so if you presently feel you are just a number at your workplace and the monotony is somewhat crushing your spirit and only a long awaited holiday or the glorious weekend can pull you through, then spend a quiet afternoon with a few fresh batches of tea or coffee and gaze at the sky. Let your mind wander, ask yourself relevant questions but most of all ask yourself what really matters! Let it sit with you and allow yourself to answer the question in a pure and honest way.

You see we all seem to reach out and hope external forces will deliver exactly what we wish to know! When deep down we already know the answers, it is your frame of mind that can distort reality and make excuses. Have you had a tightening sensation in your stomach for some time and an uneasy feeling of the mind or a scratch you just can't seem to itch? If you feel you aren't going anywhere fast and this is all your life will ever be, then you are showing much love to those around you, but not enough for yourself. Nothing happens overnight so a gradual thought process must take place, which will only serve to reinforce this new shift.

We can all change our circumstances, we just have to think the thought and once it is planted firmly then positivity will win out, the major hang up is this feeling of desire! Desire is derived from the ego, it can cause you to over control situations, furthermore it can assist you in making erroneous decisions. Because of the sheer mindless drive cast over you, it can lead you to unintentionally hurt the people around you in the process. Desire is a lustful, controlling thought, it is a yearning, it is a urging need, and it blinds you to external factors. It pushes you to stop at nothing until you achieve that goal, hence it cannot be an emotion to take lightly.

The alternative approach is to have a goal to aim for, but instead of desire in your heart and mind you should opt for hope and let optimism fill up the space, in the same way we make a wish, when we blow out the candles on a birthday cake or wish upon a shooting star. In those very moments we show our intent but we also freely give the thought out to the universe with a pure innocence. We do not try to hold onto the wish, we ask the universe for help and take great comfort from this with a quiet confidence, and so because we did not hang onto it, it also becomes lost to our conscious mind and enveloped by the subconscious.

Alan Watts asked a very important question to his students, "do you do life or does life do you?". It is only because in the past you might have asked or forced a will onto your life or another person, which played out that the dominant part of your mind thinks this ought to be the way and will continue to try to manage each situation. This is your loss of freedom! Did your life change or the result of your forced intention really play a big part? It may have even had a less than favourable outcome! Was it the cause of any friction? The influence you think you have, and the influence the universe has is of no comparison.

Life to some is a joke in which they did not fully hear, but laughed anyway. Can that realisation come too late and can we ever get to a point where we pass without regret? Yes! Regret cannot be a construct of our mind, this is the same with guilt, what happens, happens, as much as we like to think we are the builders of our own destiny and that it is us that has to repent on our actions. The things you have done and regretted in your life cannot be so as you would not have been truly mindfully aware of your actions at that time. Even if you knew there may be repercussions to the acts, this isn't being mindful this is simply trying to predict the future. When you become aware of what is, these things cannot occur with a will or without!

Everything happens for a reason, that reason might not reveal itself for some time, it does not matter if the outcome was good or if it was bad at that time, as it was a calculated synchronicity and for you to feel that it was you solely who carried this out, is a ludicrous concept.

Francis Bacon (or commonly attributed to Francis Bacon) gave us the quote "knowledge is power!" The knowledge that you ultimately know nothing is the real power! As this allows you to be open and receive what you have been searching for, we have to make mistakes so that we can expand spiritually and grow as a person. To live life trying hard to prevent ourselves from such errors is to live in fear, so if you are undamaged and unscarred by life then perhaps a question more relevant is, have I lived? Also if this existence really was heaven on earth would you experience all that is? How long before the perfect aspects start to wane a little?

As humans we rely on spontaneity, we thrive on the unknown, it makes life worth living, drama, mystery, excitement. Just like the game of chess, if it was all good and mapped out for you, you too would knock down the pieces and call the game. We require the element of surprise, good or bad it all goes towards creating a broader mind and greater endurance, if it was all great and wholesome all of the time how would we appreciate better times, to the level we can now?

In saying that, do people really appreciate the better times? As it has to be felt momentarily and they were too busy thinking of the next opportunity for happiness to come along. Another side to this is, if someone you meet is overly friendly or nice we get the sense this isn't a genuine person, they may possibly have an ulterior motive! Whether rightly or wrongly our minds cannot compute situations that feel too wholesome and tranquil or if we do we are stuck in a perpetual fear of the wheels falling off.

We should try to take things at face value in these times and cherish what is, not what will be, as this is just a figment of our imagination, a balance always, and that balance does not necessarily have to be 50/50. A scale is still in balance if leaning towards one side slightly, let that side be the side of good for that is the most powerful side, it is the side of light as opposed to dark. If you were to enter a darkroom with only a flicker of candlelight the room would still illuminate but to wish to go into a lit room holding a piece of vantablack could not be hoped to have the same desirable effect.

Make friends with the present and allow the future to tell its own story, it is true we have many surrounding factors that all contribute to the landscape of our journey, our friends and family, bosses, work colleagues, even work commitments, the debt we find ourselves in, that lead to many considerations, burdens and responsibilities, other people's greed, their opinions, control, our genetics, our predispositions to illness and disease and disabilities. When we are in relationships we have to consider our partner's points of view, likes and dislikes and how we spend our time sharing the load, unless you alter the many preconceptions you have through therapy mainly hypnosis it can feel impossible to change your ways.

Back to the question "do you do life or does life do you?". Whatever you answer may be, the point of the question isn't to shock, the answer is irrelevant. The only follow up should be, does it really matter if your answer is a firm yes? Then you have missed a valuable lesson, and the ever-present friend might just be shouting the answer for you.

The human mind can be filled with self-importance, this causes people to create friction and turmoil as a result. The only way we can grow is to remain non-judgemental, and stay humble, only when it is you that apologises first does the quarrelling subside, isn't that the point? Isn't that a positive influence we can all have! Making light of a bad situation no matter how enormous it may appear on the surface can bring about a difference in the perspective. Sometimes you might have witnessed passive aggressive behaviour from the people around you, a peculiar thing often seems to occur, humour prevails! Although the point might have been very well portrayed the comedic aspect of the gesture shines through, and the devil on the shoulder appears to go into hiding. This is a beautiful thing and something which can lift daily stresses and modern pressures in certain situations, it can have a dousing effect, a wet blanket on the fire so to speak.

The self-importance part of our being is very much on show most of the time, even in a subtle way it is still hard to conceal entirely. If a person starts a conversation more often than not with the word "I" he/she will undoubtedly have egotistical tendencies. The literary Latin translation of I is Ego, when you single yourself out with I you sort to go it alone! When we say "we", we bring a collective community aspect to the story in a modestly natured kind of way. It is very rare we can say with absolute certainty it was "I" that did said task! As we have found out your influence on any situation is limited, only with the masses can we hope to make a difference.

The seven deadly sins

In Christianity or any other religion with an adaptation of the seven deadly sins, they are meant as an avoidance in order to live a coordinated and balanced existence and for the most part their interpretations seem pretty self-evident. So let's just touch on a few that seem less obvious and look at why they were included.

Pride – why, when we are told from an early age or how proud our parents are of you, is it then classified as a deadly sin? The simple answer is, although not malicious in nature and of no perilous effect, it can deceive our sensibility. It is solely ego driven and can act and serve as an overshadowing cloaking effect on the very actions and goals we set ourselves.

The other two that seem less heinous in nature are Gluttony and Sloth, their inclusion is directly linked to our own mortality. The rest of the list has obvious unsavoury characteristics, but what is most apparent is that they are a guide in order for you to live a long and prosperous life, and each and every one is governed by the subconscious, so nothing new there then. On the one hand we find it near impossible to fight this side of our mind and its partner holding its corner. In contrast to the seven deadly sins we have the seven heavenly virtues. Also self-explanatory they are quite literally polar opposites in meaning and are as follows: Chastity – Lust, Temperance -Gluttony, Charity - Greed, Diligence - Sloth, Patience -Wrath, Kindness - Envy and finally Humility – Pride. Therefore when we show one side of this tangible duo we dispel the other and the balance can be readdressed, and so pure resolution will always win over immoral thought. Also we might try to address this balance indifference by counter action, when we try to defeat the monster, we invariably sort to become that very thing.

Advocates for equal rights in regards to racism, feminism or a completely different category namely climate change, understandably and commendably seek change after bearing witness to appalling travesties, which have and are still very much apparent in the world today. However, sometimes their yearning for change or ways to help in a situation may be blighted by misdirection, in circumstances they don't fully understand. In certain cases this can exacerbate the problem further. "There! There! You'll be okay now!" said the monkey placing a fish safely up a tree.

We can focus on the wrong things and so use up vital energy and effort at the wrong time or interval, this is not to say we shouldn't seek to correct the course of such doings but it is in the manner that we present ourselves and the task in hand that is the key. Climate change, a popular topic of recent times with carbon footprints and the decimation of our natural global resources, is without doubt a very worthy cause and should be at the forefront of global leaders' agendas.

Ways are already being implemented to counteract this humanistic self-induced destruction of the earth, with alternative approaches. But maybe all that is needed is the spread of awareness and mindful action at the right times, the next part might sound counter intuitive, but the best piece of advice that can be given and not just in relation to this impending issue, but also in everyday life with the many mistakes we make, whether singularly or collectively, this advice being to "sit on our hands" you may ask, but nothing will get done and so nothing will change! Very true in a momentary sense, but what is widely accepted as the biggest healer?

Of course time! time is only a concept and has no real actual evidence for its reality, but it is by far the greatest advocate for change and for undoing all that is done. Take one of the biggest man made catastrophes the world has seen, the Chernobyl Nuclear power plant explosion. A monumental, disaster with extreme repercussions and yet here we are 30-plus years later, with all the global predictions about the environment, now we see nature reclaiming what was rightfully hers and animals returning to what was. Yes the radiation levels are still extremely high in certain parts, but something as simple as the wildlife and fauna returning so soon speaks volumes and gives hope to all circumstances. It is not idle to sit on your hands, it is absolutely imperative at times to do so! In that way we do not prolong the issue. Our incessant need for control can quickly escalate errors we have made, instead of demanding, show the compassion you so sorely seek, for only then can you make that very change happen, it is all relative, but it is all subjective and so, all circumstantial.

Family, friendships and companionships

At times through the year we start to become more aware of those around us, seasonal festivities, times of good cheer and bringing good unto others. But as quickly as it comes it is all soon forgotten, why? Because on those occasions the stresses of life, the eternal juggling act has a momentary interval? Because it is a time for charitable giving or helping others? Or is it because we get a brief chance to see exactly what it feels like to live in the present and focus our attention on this reality? It is all of these things! This is what life is really all about, shared memories, time for appreciation of the very things we already have.

This book is designed as a gentle tap on the shoulder, a soft whisper in the ear, to serve as a small reminder of what the truly important things in life are, a simple awareness check to dispel the myth of the search for the Holy Grail of just what it is to feel alive and our approach to life! Family, friendships, relationships, our collective companionships, the very connection we feel when we are with those close to us. It is the embodiment of our nature, the warmth you see in your family's eyes, a sense of closeness, the shared experiences, times for celebrations, tribulations. A curious thing is that once connected and a closeness is achieved with something or somebody, we begin to feel both their joy and pain on an intimate level. That is reality, strange occurrences bring thought provoking ideas. For instance Couvade Syndrome, this is more often referred to as sympathy pains a husband or partner may feel it as a direct pain attributed to what their pregnant partner is feeling, but can also bring about feelings of envy or guilt for either their partner being able to become pregnant or the fact it was them who participated in the act this resulting pain.

When our parents, siblings or children are going through a traumatic episode we do not just share the anguish but we physically go through the same pain as if our own hearts were breaking or that our bodies are going through the same emotional or physical endurance. The connective mirroring effect is visible to see, it is unbiased. Whether good or bad. Life is life there can be no need to complicate this matter further. Blood of course is thicker than water, you can change your friends but you can't change your family, they share our hopes and ambitions, they teach us about life and of ourselves, they share our genetics, you will never feel an instant connection like you do with your family.

So relationships, what is the criteria in an intimate relationship? Shared interests, similar beliefs, morality, humour? In a nutshell, likeminded people! But the paradox is we wish to also find someone unique, who is different and can offer a different lifestyle to our own stagnant existence, opposites attract. However, they also have to hold the same values and similar traits our own next of kin possess, a woman may perhaps in the back of her mind try to find endearing qualities shown by her father in a new suitor, same with a man, he may want to gain the warmth and affection shown by his mother. But ultimately we try to find ourselves in others and a bond is created, sometimes for a lifetime. We become so intimate that we can begin to know what the other person is thinking. We can end up becoming so in sync with our partner we start to finish off each other's sentences. Relationships are a control aspect to our life, we risk pain for love. We can choose just who they are, we see external beauty in others yet the beauty within seems not quite as important when commencing a relationship.

Many starting a coupling suffer the negatives because of the aesthetics, this may be instinctual or attraction via hormonal scent and genetic paring, a good match physically but not mentally or spiritually. If we feel it maybe a little too one sided we can opt to close the book on that chapter and move on! What we cannot do is simply try to domineer that person or vice versa, though many feel the need to do so and that it is their right, therefore a change is very much sought after in the partner.

Once again with temperamental consequences the overcritical entity has popped back up out of obscurity. The strangest thing we find is that the aspects we fault in others are usually the things we most fear and are aware of in ourselves. This is a fight we should never wish to participate in, if it feels like tremendous effort to control the circumstances maybe that in itself should serve to enlighten you. People often stay in relationships for longer than they should, even when the obvious dynamics are just not working. We fight and argue based on our emotions instead of acting with mindfulness, our own importance takes over and a clash follows suit, a needless waste of your spiritual energy. This also drains our bodies in the process. We are who we are and the only person who can and ought to change that is ourselves, so living a lie to please others isn't harmonious cohabitation, it is a consequentially futile endeavour to force that which cannot be forced. This goes for friendships too, even though your overwhelming mind is telling you 'yes but you love them' this is a sinister promise that can muddy the waters, also coupled with it telling you 'others will think bad of you' or 'you might not be able to get anyone better'. This all has the desired effect of causing fear and a prolonging of the agony as a result.

Yes we are all beautiful, we are all one but the other person's awareness of that fact may be lacking and so the synchronised harmony we sought for in the pairing will be left wanting, you have to learn to love yourself before another and what is rightfully due for you will come to be. You might be accustomed to a solitary life, or on a break in which you are trying to discover who you are and what you really want out of life, once you get a clearer picture of this you will stand in better stead on this love topic. Marital or civil relationships do not have the same solidarity and meaning they once did. Not in every case, but for the most part the symbolism of unity has lost a great deal of its power in recent times and that might be okay as civilisation progresses. Our adaptability has to also change - female liberation, equal rights at home and in the workplace - among many other settings. The dynamics of a relationship have altered tremendously with this most righteous of acts, a sway to androgynous times might be in the balance and a readdress of the boundaries. The only negative of the recent era is our incessant need for perfection within the unity, it is far easier without the 1950's frowns to leave or even cheat on a partner than to work through life's problems. 'Plenty of fish in the sea' and so is the case, if something is not right then no amount of hard work will change that fact. The tables have been turned within the roles of our feminine and masculine traits. For millennia we knew the male role was to provide, to be the breadwinner and protect - the quintessential hunter gatherer archetype. It is true men still have vestigial traits from times gone by or what is considered by the opposing sex as pathological aspects to the male species. Now with the much needed equality within the workplace and vastly changing career options, manly pride may have taken a tumble and this has bred insecurities.

We now see in certain age groups women who, although extremely successful and powerful in other roles, have started to use their sexuality and prowess increasingly in acquiring gain or a longed for relationship, compared to the decades of the '30s and '40s in which women were given a ridiculous fine if they showed so much as a thigh on the beach. As an observing officer would carry a tape measure to see how long or short the women's bathing costumes were. Now it is a form of liberation and rightly so, as there can never be one rule for one and one rule for another. For the most part our evolution was a gradual process, however, over the last few centuries the lives we live have proceeded ahead of our adaptations. It is a fine balancing act, it was always an unfair assumption that the stronger of the species got to be the protector, show dominance over the other, but for the longest time that is how it was, as mirrored by the animal kingdom. We should be mindful of this moving forward not to berate others but to show understanding. At times we miss the beat when it comes to careful considerations. It is true, times have changed and those changes are always for the better, but we should not force our adaptability, it will simply happen when nature intends it to. So what about other companionships we seek out, namely animals, our beautifully affectionate pets? It doesn't matter what animal we choose they all have the same effect, they save us from our loneliness, help us through hard times and show us love unconditionally or show stability for a family. A lot can be learnt from this most innocent of connections, the most popular pets being cats and dogs.

An often dividing question we have when coming into contact with a person for the first time is, "are you a dog person or a cat person?" Both can show ample amounts of affection to lift our mood. They can behave childlike, can have hissy fits but without a glimmer of malice only an instinctual reactions, a pet can centre a family, teach children responsibilities, help with anxiety, shower you with their doting attention and it poses the question, do we really deserve them at times? Only through the most fortunate of circumstances. Nature, the great outdoors, our surrounding environment. What comes to mind at the mere mention of the word nature? Is it a luscious green forest, a beautiful valley on a mountainside? The silky shimmer of seasonal spring grass or the birds in the trees singing their specific melodies? Nature is life, it has a way of calming people like no other. It can instil serenity and lift our spirits with a connection so strong we cannot put an adequate name on it. From hearing the morning calls of the blackbirds to the clicks of bats in the night, nature helps humanity feel an unbreakable bond with this planet.

We are so busy living at times we forget just how much of a positive effect it has on our soul. Taking our shoes and socks off to walk on the grass between the hanging branches of a tree, not only nurtures our mental wellbeing but also grounds our electrical bodies, removing any pent up restless energy and connects our body directly to where it came from.

Watching a sunrise, sunset or looking straight up at the cosmos in the night sky can give you an enormous feeling of belonging and allows the soul to orate openly without impairment. In contrast to all the beauty that we find around us, there are many acts of violence shown too – from tsunamis, tornadoes, volcanic eruptions and bushfires to global pandemics which can decimate a significant part of the human population. Why? This question arises when they either directly influence our circumstances or we observe the pain and suffering of others on the global news broadcasts. It can be a bitter pill to swallow and cause someone to feel disdain for the situation.

We ask soul searching questions and even question our own religious beliefs. If there really is a God then why would they permit such despicable and deplorable events to happen? Everything physical we are is the result of the most violent series of events imaginable - from the big bang, star formations, and cosmic collisions to unfathomable elementary explosions.

Take our very own little blue planet for instance, everything around we see is down to many colossal impacts, tremendous amounts of heat, violence, electrical storms even the air we breathe and the water we drink to survive came to be as a result of this, asteroids and smaller comets carrying vast amounts of ice crashing into our precious sapphire entwined emerald gemstone. Indeed our very existence can be credited to these very facts.

Life and death

The sombre topic of death! Given the choice for immortality on this planet you could hazard a guess as high as 90 to 95% of people would opt out if they really thought about it, this is due to the fact that fundamentally most people know there is a time to leave this world. The only problem that arises is that the time in their minds may differ significantly from reality. Achieving their goals etc, it may possibly feel as though we are asked to leave the party just as the music is about to start. This is where the unease of death lies.

If we are told we have a terminal illness or feel able bodied enough in the latter stages of our life a universally accepted list is sometimes compiled, the inspirational bucket list! A strong and heroic deed for anyone to see through with all they are having to endure, it is with the utmost merit these people see out their lifelong wish list of experiences. The only possible downside that can be seen with this list is, why do we wait for our calling before setting our sights on such things? A puzzlement of complexities there can be no doubt! The main reason is we become so busy planning our future we neglect the present and only when such serious events come to the forefront do we start to ask 'what are the really important things?' 'What do I actually want from this life?' It should not take a prolific event for you to experience and analyse this provocative thought. The most apt examination of your life should be why aren't you fulfilling such things now? The funerals of friends and family are seen as marked macabre times were we are often left grief stricken by the loss and although we are told we should not be upset and that we should instead celebrate their life, it is of course a period spent with mixed emotions. Sadness is felt consciously but kept in our unconscious mind, for it knows it will have to live without this familiar constant. It is true we ought to celebrate each life for they have achieved greatness, they have suffered profusely and come through it all with a sense of spiritual dignity.

Gurus

These specific self-proclaimed guides to enlightenment profess to having such wisdom that they can reveal answers to questions we have often pondered. The so-called gurus ask many to listen to their teachings, and in return grant their followers access to the true meaning of life! Yet they already know the answer resides within their subjects. A main stay of their existence in this field comes in how profound they can make a quote feel, most new age life teachers more than likely spend the better part of a day maybe even a week coming up with a pithy, witty turn of phrase, usually an obvious statement shrouded in cryptic mystery, and then present it to their adorning fans in public or on social media! It is easy to see why they try to out rank one another. It can be difficult to identify and take in the meanings of said quotes, when they themselves do not seem to practice what they preach, they build a lifestyle on keeping the answers close to their chest, letting snippets of the truth out one by one. It would be more efficient for them to say, "look inside for what you seek, that is where the fountain of knowledge exists". They hold nothing special you don't already have, their trick is to get you to believe that they do! Like a magician who never reveals their secrets, you can fleece a sheep many times but you can only skin it once, to enlighten somebody once is a gracious thing but to ask them to keep returning can be just plain cruel.

The Dalai Lama gives freely, he shows his modest ways, he does not wish to be glorified, his only wish is to spread his message of awareness, a beautifully kind and generous entity, but many others seem to want to build fan bases and acquire wealth from the very people they are trying to help. If you wish to become famous and popular via the masses of followers who look up to you, how can you then be expected to be taken seriously when your message is about shunning pride and egotistical ways? It is certainly food for thought, they challenge you with guidance such as "try to be the best version of yourself" and that seems pretty straight forward, so we go off and take this message to heart and become mindful of it in our actions, but we try too hard and it becomes a real struggle because we feel we are on a constant guilt trip. Might it not be wiser to first come to terms with and understand exactly what is the best version of ourselves? Only then can we ultimately and effortlessly become that person. We are meant to have and show these emotions instilled in us for better and for worse, the good, the bad and the ugly. The gurus we listen to have profound knowledge and we like to associate and attach ourselves to such poetic and meaningful citations, they say so little but mean so much. We treat them as guides for our own self-help, but sometimes their objectives can be intriguing, constructing evocative sentiments can go some way in helping people understand hidden meanings and that might be just what is required in times of need or when we lose our way, but to purposefully formulate sayings just to come across as profound and of the utmost intelligence, can sometimes sit uneasy on the mind as opposed to transparent teachings.

The words in this book only serve to gently remind you of the things you already know, at the times we have wandered astray of the path and in our perceived reality. Gurus live tranquil existences and have found meaning and insight through their practices. If they can spread hope and awareness with their joyful messages, then the positives outweigh the negatives. We have to be wary of the trap though. Most messages are quite self-explanatory with an obvious premise, but as they are told by a gentle, passive, well natured being in a faintly veiled poetic way, it catches our imagination and they can become idols, it can also help them achieve that very status and lifestyle they deem much more befitting of themselves.

A book you may have heard of, but let's change the title slightly, let's call it *Mortality* subheading reads *A book for all those who will die*. That is quite an abundant audience you have to agree and let's pluck out a random quote from another of life's guru's work and see if you become enlightened by it, 'the quieter you become, the more you can hear'. The underlining message meaning that when we quieten our minds from all of the chatter, the clearer we can hear our true thoughts! Each and every quote seems to follow suit, some maybe a little harder to understand with subtle cryptic clues 'The ultimate power that many modern gurus offer is false hope. Their programs calling us to unlimited power have made them rich, not us. They touch our false selves and tap our toxic shame' John Bradshaw. We search outwardly for answers each and every day, whether that be from acquaintances, intellects or gurus, when it was ourselves that held the key all along. This may all seem quite judgemental and a deformation of certain characters, but it is just meant as a simple, humorous yet passively aggressive way of delivering a message.

The false prophets make careers from the fallen, they are allowed to live a pleasant existence as it is facilitated by the very people they claim to aid. We too would also be at peace in similar circumstances, but the normality of the average person is far removed from that. Their message should be unequivocally relayed so that it can be construed without hesitation, a clear and concise meaning for all to comprehend. The Buddha (Siddhartha Gautama) did not wish to be idolised, he too gave his message freely; Buddhism is seen as a religion, but it truly is a way of life, you might have possibly heard the story of the young Prince Siddhartha whose mother died giving birth to him. Stricken with heartbreak and anguish his kingly father ordered that the young prince remained at all times within the confines of the palace walls, with every luxury imaginable so as to not leave him wanting for anything.

This became the only life he knew, this was the king's way of trying to save his son from any pain and suffering. The reason was also that at only a few days old a holy man prophesied over the young prince (although some accounts acknowledge 9 brahman holy men made the prophecy). He proclaimed that the young child would either grow up to be a great ruler or a great spiritual leader.

Through Siddhartha's childhood his great king father made every effort to hide any religious texts or teachings from his son as a way to lean the prophecy to that of a great ruler. So a most tranquil and joyous life was led by the young prince. But by the age of 20 his curiosity had played with him long enough and he asked his closest confidante to show him life outside the palace walls. Once outside he became perplexed as to the wailing and suffering all around. One time, he asked his friend and king's guard, "Why is that man dancing so strangely and what has become of his hair?". The guard replied, "That man is not dancing, he's frail of foot and also weak so cannot walk the same as you or me! And his hair has lost its body and colour for he is old." Right then the prince saw a funeral procession and enquired about it. His friend said that the man had passed over and his family were on their way to bury him. The prince remarked, "Do we all grow old and die?" "Yes it is a part of life my friend." This sudden realization alarmed the prince and he wanted to return to the confines of the palace immediately. A short time had passed and the prince bore a child but his heart and mind was so unsettled he felt compelled to leave in order to seek the truth of life, and so he left in the dead of night. He spent his first two years of self-induced exile in meditation under the guidance of two spiritual teachers and learned to be still with his thoughts. After this, he wandered the land for more answers, meeting many others like him also on the same quest. Most of the people he met told him the way to seek the truth laid in resisting the very thing they desired most, one abstained from sleep, another from speech, one from warmth and comfort and so on. They all asked him what his likes were and his response was food as he felt he was constantly hungry. "There is your answer," they replied and so he spent the next six months in a permanent state of starvation only coming to eat three sesame seeds at the end. But after months of suffering he realised he was no closer to the truth and started to eat as normal, much to the dismay of the others.

So on he went on his journey. Finally arriving at the bodhi tree, he proclaimed to himself, "You shall not leave the shade of this tree till you have found the enlightenment you are searching for". Mara came to him, the mind's enemy who seeks to tempt and destroy. First he sent his beautiful daughters to tempt and distract him and said, "get him to desire you," for Mara knew that if he found enlightenment he would tell others, so the Buddha (Siddhartha) had to find that moment of stillness again. But Mara persisted and made him feel the full force of his army, he proclaimed, "be plagued by your worst nightmares". This caused much self-doubt and he asked himself, "are you sure you have what it takes to achieve Nirvana? Are you worthy enough?". But as he touched the earth, the earth spoke, "he is worthy!" and Siddhartha saw his hundreds of past lives. And saw how what he had done in one life influenced the next, he saw life as a wheel, some always moving upwards, whilst others always falling downwards. Birth, death and rebirth, and the three poisons, hate, greed and stupidity that kept the wheel turning! He came to the conclusion whether your life is easy or hard the one thing you can't escape is death. But suddenly what he had been searching for was revealed to him, if he did not fear death and accepted this truth! Death had no power thus came the knowledge that in order to avoid or save oneself from suffering was to free yourself from wanting anyone or anything (no attachment). To be ready always to give and receive, and in that moment, Buddha had found what he was searching for, that elusive enlightenment (awakening). "You see you do not need the luxuries of life and also you are not required to cause yourself harm through sacrifices, you should travel down the middle road only then will you find the meaning of life!" And so on the forty ninth day it finally came to him after Mara had sent his plague he also started to relive a childhood memory of a game he had been a spectator to.

Whilst watching the ploughing tournaments he realised although the rest of the crowd cheered and revelled in the games, all he could see was death and suffering from the insects being trampled to the sweat and anguish on the competitors' faces, and so it dawned on him that he need not to try to cause himself pain and suffering, and he did not require any of life's luxuries! Therefore he needed to just be, without desire! This is a way to avoid self-induced pain and achieve spiritual growth. When we desire something or decide how things ought to be, we set ourselves up for a fall. We're trying to dictate each aspect of our life and the circumstances around us, in turn causing ourselves untold pain and mental anguish in the process. Life is life and as soon as that is understood and accepted you are free and at peace with it. Desire is control and it starts to become pretty obvious who the perpetrator is. There are three ways of life that we can all incorporate into our own paths, one is Buddhism, one is stoicism and lastly we have Taoism. There is no need for any extremes or to expel any effort amongst these three practices, all that is required is an awareness and understanding of the principles, then can you harness their practices to enhance your experience with a majestic flow.

A brief insights into stoicism - founded by Zeno of Citium in the 3rd century BC Athens, it is a philosophy, a train of thought. The logic is very similar to Buddhism, but instead of the concepts of Nirvana or enlightenment it has Eudaimonia, meaning happiness or blessedness. It also holds desire in contempt as the principle player underlining all of humanity's suffering. It states 'we should accept the moment as it presents itself and have no presumptions of how it ought to be'. Stoicism believes virtue is the only good and that materialistic possessions, pleasure, health and wealth are not intrinsically good nor bad, but have a value in which virtues can act upon. Certain emotions are believed to result from errors of judgement and we ultimately should aim to maintain a will. A person's actions show that individual's resolution and philosophy, it is not their words. The biggest and best serving of the stoic teaching resides in the control, non-control aspects of life, as the things out of our hands cannot be fretted over and should not cause anxiety. When we show emotion to outside forces we are controlled by them. When we believe and accept this we can truly detach our minds from such occurrences.

Why get angry at someone's actions? Because it directly affects you, right? But how? Because you lost control of the situation and that can result in a hardship. Our senses create our reality, or more to the point our interpretation of the senses creates the reality in our minds. If a negative force or influence comes into contact with you is there a way of altering your reactions? Yes, it is very simple, accept it and cherish it, learn from it but never be governed by it. To show emotions at negative circumstances is futile and will only serve to prolong the agony. The only real influence you can hope to have originates with you and your mind, as with life there will be encounters that are less favourable but it is up to you to stay or to leave the scenario or adapt your behaviour in a way that changes the circumstances.

When we feel the victim we become the victim, when we do not react, there cannot be any continuance of the action. Go within at these times and remind yourself what is important, will this have any lasting effect? Will it even be a memory? Just because something feels important at that very moment does make is so. Is it your self-pride that is hurt or the loss of power that is causing this turmoil? Learn to understand what you can influence and what you cannot and allow the buck to rest there.

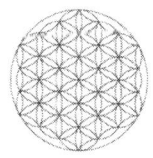

SYNCHRONICITIES

Carl Jung, the Analytical Psychologist, not only gave us the concept of the shadow, our subconscious hidden self, but also theorised that synchronicities were events of 'meaningful coincidence' if they occur but have no causal relationship that seems to be meaningfully related. It can also relate to certain numbers and symbols that spring up in our lives but hold an interpretable relevance to each of us. Read this description carefully: 'the coincidental occurrences of events and especially psychic events (as similar thoughts and widely separated persons or a mental image of an unexpected events before it happens) that seem related but are not explained by conventional mechanisms of causality'. Déjà vu, Karma, chance, fate, good fortune, bad fortune, omens, wishes, intuition, sixth sense, superstition, negativity and positivity can all be encompassed by this term. We say to ourselves and others "everything happens for a reason" or "isn't it funny how things work out?" when things go in our favour, but question why when they don't, because our logical minds cannot fathom how seemingly random meaningful acts come to be. So we call it a mere coincidence and draw a line under it. So is there more to this than we dare to contemplate?

Throughout history we have categorised certain superstitions, songs, fables and tall tales. Throughout human civilization these types of stories may have been created to explain peculiar circumstances and in this way our negative self attributes bad occurrences to happenings foretelling the future. We see magpies and salute to stave off the unlucky omen or sing the song to find out if a positive maybe bestowed onto us if there are more than one in sight. Avoiding cracks on the pavement, being careful not to break a mirror, a black cat crossing our path, not walking under a ladder, beginner's luck or keeping a lucky rabbit's foot (although not very lucky for the rabbit) universal numbers also play a part. The number 666 is credited with being the so-called sign of the devil, the number 323 is said to be an angelic number.

You will have heard the saying "good and bad things come in threes". Nikola Tesla stated, "if only you knew the magnificence of the numbers three, six and nine then you would hold the key to the universe". Mind, body and spirit, the pathways that force energy/information to manifest into material form. You may have a lucky number of your own. Asian countries also hold specific numbers in high regard, to signify certain phenomena, traits of good and bad fortune, to show prosperity and also failure. So, what can this all mean, do synchronicities actually have any significance to our lives? The short answer is, undoubtedly yes! But that would be an easy get out, wouldn't you agree? So let us peel back the outer layers to this perplexing notion, just as to plant a seed in the topsoil is to plant a thought in the mind.

How many times have you woke up on the wrong side of bed and proceeded to have an awful start to the day? Burnt toast, spilt coffee down your nice new top, to forgetting where you left the car keys and as a result become slightly late leaving for work and then of course it's just your luck that you end up stuck behind a slow driver! Then frustration kicks in with the realisation that your slight lateness is turning into a possible disciplinary at work, and to top it off the traffic lights conspire against you and instantly turn to red on your immediate approach. At this point you are totally controlled by your unconscious mind in your actions. It is only the conscious mind that can feel this chaos and anger and your whole character is altered at that very moment. Road rage, the descension of the red mist are both terms given to describe this exact event. You feel you are more important than any other driver and because of the safety of your car you start to display your utter contempt for the other road user, something you couldn't even imagine portraying face to face in the street.

The only way real to change these circumstances is to simply become aware of just what elements are at play here, then purposefully proceed to change the environment and also your focus, opening the car window to let in a soothing breeze, turning on the radio or changing to a calmer station or if extremely irritable pulling the car over for five minutes to reflect. You are late anyway and so whether that be twenty or twenty-five minutes really isn't going to change the prevailing outcome. What is the really important thing here? The pressures you have put on yourself are unjust! What has just happened will be forgotten within a week or two and so it really shouldn't matter at that precise moment. Mindful awareness is the key, this instantaneously eases the mind, it might even cause a smile and laughter at the misfortune gifted to you that very morning. Most importantly, it will help to centre you and return you efficiently and comfortably back to the present, essentially pulling your mind out of that illusionary future, in which you were being held captive, with irrational thoughts of:

- "My boss is going to be mad"
- "I'm supposed to be at such in such place"
- "I've let people down"
- "I'm not a good person for not keeping my word"

which are wholly self-critical and brought on solely by our tormentor and only serve to magnify, escalate the nightmarish circumstances. Now let us look at the days in which you have woken up early and fresh after a peaceful night's rest. You have time for a nice long bath or shower, you may have even been able to carry out some exercise or took the dog for a walk, iron your clothes, made your hair presentable, ate a wholesome breakfast, you could have had time to read the newspaper or listen to the news and voila! You are in your car 10 minutes earlier than usual so no need to rush to get to work today. In fact you take a little extra time on the road that morning so that you do not arrive too early. You listen to your favourite album, the sun has just popped out from behind the clouds, the road is clear and to top it off every traffic light senses your presence and jumps instantly to green and it can feel like you are being given the keys to the city. Are you feeling stressed in this scenario, is your anxiety flaring, do you actually feel relaxed and happy with an overwhelming positivity ready to receive the day ahead? Quite possibly! You see, you get back what you give out, it is the universal law otherwise known as karma.

Many people class this under the same category as superstition, and something that should not be taken too seriously. As once you deny it, is to also plead ignorance, we cannot possibly believe wholeheartedly that karma is a real thing with substance and so we disregard it and see it as immaterial, but that is the denier working hard to get you to come to that presumption. This has little to do with faith. It may not be in perfect balance to our timescale but balance in time there is no doubt. There are two convergences taking place at all times, one is our own collective consciousness and the other is universal will. Nothing is meaningless, everything plays its own little part whether in our own story or the story of the cosmos, and to dispute this is to dispute our very existence.

Many don't allow themselves to see synchronicities or happenings from the intent of the universe as this would cause a mental loss of control and fear from our egotistical self. So onto the other side, do you have an influence on these events? The answer is a unanimous yes! Your good and bad vibes, the positive and negative energy we keep referring to, what we give out we receive, this energy is real. If you find yourself faced with an argument where the facts are misted and so you proceed to face this head on and stand your corner, as attack is the best form of defence, therefore a blazing row ensues. When met with hostility we tense, we grit our teeth and continue to create a false front in order to protect ourselves, fighting fire with fire in theory can work as this act stifles the oxygen. The trouble is we lose our essence in the process, this returns us to the stoic quote of Marcus Aurelius 'receive without pride, let go without attachment'. But we carry on arguments mainly to protect that very pride.

So what could have been a discussion in which the truth was revealed turns to hate as reflection occurs. This is the mirroring effect, if we are unsure of what or who is right or even if we are sure then a simple and genuinely put across "okay" will immediately douse the flames and cause what seemed a very much important stance to be laughed off. It was the conscious attention that prolonged the quarrel partly due to each party having that sinister being whisper doubt in their ears. When times are hard and you seem to never catch a break, it is you and you only that can change this cycle. And the easiest way? Is to lose the "I" lose that self-importance and change your own outlook, interpret struggles as lessons in growth, appreciate all the good vibrations instead of continuing to see the hardships. Picture yourself at the centre of a circle looking outwardly at the world, the slightest shifts in either direction could completely change the observable landscape, bringing fresh, new ideas and perspectives into focus, casting a new light hence transforming your own outlook on life. This is to show there need not be an almighty change for a difference to be felt deep in the mind. The universe is unbiased, things happen and they should never be taken too personal. You have the power to influence this! so, maybe having that in your locker with a quiet confidence is all that's needed in relieving what seems to be the more persistently stagnated aspects to your existence! inspiring you with a new found vibrance to search for inspirational therefore eternal and meaningful discoveries, giving you a better understanding of who you really are ! irrespective of your prior circumspect approach.

Form the habit of giving out positive vibrations and watch how things start to unfold. It will come as no surprise that life will reshuffle the deck and everything you are and the newly found actions you have taken will receive an abundance of positivity in return. Trust in the universe, never seek revenge or retribution as two wrongs will never make a right as the universal law will never grant that wish. Never intently wish bad karma onto others, for by doing so well! you can gather what will come of this! Trust this to happen but never desire it to be so with envy and jealousy in your heart.

As mentioned, there are stark contrasts between a wish and desire. You may make a wish when you are fortunate enough to witness the mesmerising sight of a meteorite breaking through the earth's upper atmosphere. The main thing we are taught is to keep those wishes a secret, another superstitious trait, and you throw out that wish with total abandon to the powers of the cosmos with hope in your heart confidently knowing you will play a very little part in the coming truths of such a wish, but feel happy there could be a possibility of it happening. This has a naturally acquired uplifting effect, it is a lesson as to how we should live our life, trust in the process, have hope in your heart and never sweat the small stuff. Be kind to others, isn't that the message? Look at when we desire something, desire is fraught with dominance. Do you find the more you desire something the more that very thing appears to elude you, forever moving further from your grasp? But there is a correlation, as great things can sometimes happen unexpectedly. This is all down to the fact that our lustful focus wasn't on the gain or of obtaining it. We sometimes say, "well that was an unexpected bit of good fortune" after a windfall in times of need. We ask ourselves and others what our deepest, darkest desires are! in this very question we answer the narrative, it is soaked in futile negativity and becomes something we shouldn't hope to succeed in. This is not to say we should not have goals in our lives or hope that our wishes come true, but that in the same way the universe shows with an aim, a will and a fundamental direction, we should throw caution to the wind and give the power over to the 'Tao'. To try to hold onto the reins is to hold onto life with the same grip of tension and fear, be at one with it, allow it to work for and with you as opposed to causing head on collisions at every turn, Think the thought, set the wheels in motion and enjoy the ride! for you are the passenger on this explicit journey and not the chauffeur. When you wish, the wish does not stay with you indefinitely, it is cast out to the world and forgotten by the mind - this is how dreams come true! How often have you experienced déjà vu? Is this strange phenomena the result of a previous dream state in which a glimmer of the future had been foretold? Is it a memory of a memory, an echo of a past life crossing over to our own reality or just a simple illusion of the mind.

Fate, the universe tells you daily, it shows you the good and bad. It may seem subtle but it is still very much there to see! unless you have fell regrettably blind by your own ignorance. Whilst many believe that all of this is just random acts of insignificance, how many things need to be revealed before it feels too compelling to simply disregard such events? Once this is classed as bad luck, good luck or even magical nonsense by a person then the blinkers have become firmly attached to that individual. Why do some believe things happen for a reason and some think it is all aimless spontaneity that could never be explained? One possible explanation for this is that some people believe because they have witnessed something so unexplainable in their life it would seem foolish not to. Do you think the contrary and become ushered into this belief system? For the majority of people who come to this conclusion, it is as a result of going within to seek the answer.

Meditation and pineal gland stimulation

The growing trend in meditation in the western world is unprecedented in recent times. What can this be attributed to? The increasing pace of life, society and culture has brought upon the populous over the last few decades? An increase to our awareness through the many easily accessible mediums, namely technology and the internet? What can be gained through the practice of meditation and why has it become so popular across the divide of eastern and western cultures? Many reading this may already be avid meditators and will be accustomed to the plethora of benefits it can and does offer. All with different intentions and all at different stages of enlightenment. Some might have initially started to meditate as a way of lifting the daily stresses and form personal relaxation techniques to carry on through, whilst others had a curiosity to open the box of Zen spirituality. Everyone who has taken up meditation will in some way achieve a spiritual awakening, this will only be enhanced by repetitious practice. Whatever the reason, meditation is an immensely helpful and powerful tool to use and can serve as our very own metronome for life, essentially steadying the ship, the benefits it has shown on a scientific level (although maybe not fully corroborated but understood to be) are, firstly, stress reduction. It has a significant way of reducing cortisol in our bodies which in turn reduces the release of sometimes harmful chemicals known as cytokines which have inflammatory promoting qualities leaving so many noticeable ailments we have all encountered from time to time including fever, headaches, low blood pressure, rapid heartbeat, rashes (eczema, etc) nausea and even trouble breathing. Although predominately a helpful bodily response to fight infections and mediate normal cellular processes, it is the over production that causes harm brought on by stress as a normal response, it is our interpretations of stressful situations that can be our downfall.

Meditation can also help us manage our anxieties, our seemingly consistent state of anxiety at variable levels in individuals is brought on solely by fear, fear of the unknown or fear of the past replaying in the future, and so negative experiences being encountered again. It helps many to feel present again. This is one of the most beneficial traits it has to offer. As a by-product of lessening stress and centring a person it also reduces anxiety- related mental health issues, sometimes drastically. It can promote emotional health which improves self-image analysis giving a healthier, positive outlook on life which can decrease the severity of depression in certain individuals. It enhances self-awareness, allows for better concentrations to be developed, may assist in the reduction of age related memory loss, can be shown to generate kindness in the psyche, may help in the fight against addiction, and it also improves sleep quality, which is possibly the most highly regarded positive to come from the practice as this directly helps humanity experience the reality of life at the truest level lifting our mood.

Meditation also helps control pain through understanding, awareness and acceptance. Lowering the intensity which can also reduce blood pressure making for a healthier cardiovascular system, a mighty list you'd have to agree.

So, what are the spiritual benefits of meditation? It releases emotional suppressions paving the way for a peaceful mind to be developed, it helps people to let go of the past and stop speculating about the future, it relaxes the nervous system and helps the physical body unwind so that a stronger connection with the higher self can be obtained, allowing a flow through the chakras to be achieved more easily with repetition. It slowly and comfortably helps a person realise who their truest self is, helping them to be at peace with who they are and empowering them to achieve a higher state of consciousness. The origin of meditation is somewhat up for debate. The oldest records of the practice of Dhyana in India dates to around 1500 BCE which has references to the training of the mind. As with this debate there is always much speculation to consider as the Buddha is said to have sat under the bodhi tree searching for meaning and enlightenment in a serene trance-like state around 2500 BCE. Although the oldest documented images date back as far as 3500 BCE, many of these records come from the Hindu tradition of Vedantism, another reasonable origin is found in the writings of Taoist Lao Tzu an ancient Chinese philosopher from between the 4th and 5th centuries BC.

Many differing religions and traditions have forms of meditation unique to their individual practices, but they are all at one with their goal. The variations can be many, some of the most popular being mindfulness meditation, spiritual meditation, focused meditation, movement meditation, mantra meditation and transcendental meditation. They can be guided or unguided, there can also be chakra meditation, chakra is the Sanskrit word translating to a disc or wheel. Chakra meditation involves a transfer of energy wheels throughout the body and each chakra having a different meaning and association.

The root chakra, located at the base of spine. Once you are in the lotus position it is the root chakra that grounds and centres you, allowing for a connection with the earth to brought about. It is our foundation and is said to have a connection to career, money stability, mindset, and a sense of belonging, associated with the spine, legs, arms and circulatory system.

The sacral chakra, located in the lower abdomen this is our connection and ability to accept others and new experiences. It holds properties of sexuality and pleasure, well-being and sense of abundance, associated with the immune system and detoxification system.

The solar plexus chakra, located in the upper abdomen stomach area, holds properties of personal power and the ability to channel. It is connected to self-worth and self-confidence and associated with the central nervous system, digestive tract and epidermis.

The heart chakra, located in the centre of our chest, holds properties of our ability to love, relationships, self-acceptance, emotional issues of love, joy and inner peace associated with the heart, thymus and lower lungs.

The throat chakra, located in the pit of the throat, holds properties of our ability to communicate, self-expression and the truth we speak, and is associated with the thyroid, respiratory system and vocal cords.

The third eye chakra, located between the brows, holds properties of, our ability to focus and see the wider picture, intuition, sense of purpose and direction in life, associated with the pituitary gland, pineal gland, eyes and sinuses.

The crown chakra, located at the apex, our highest chakra represents the ability to be fully connected with spirituality associated with the pineal gland, brain and nervous system.

- Root Chakra – Red – Mujadara
- Sacral Chakra – Orange – Svadhistitha
- Solar Plexus Chakra – Yellow – Manipura
- Heart Chakra – Green – Anuhata
- Throat Chakra – Blue – Vishuddha
- Third Eye Chakra – Indigo – Anja
- Crown Chakra – Violet – Sahasrara

The aim of the chakras is to find the balance of each entity wheel. The way we observe and focus our attention is the way we can find harmony between each one.

Now going back to meditation, the aim isn't to go into meditation with a will to achieve, the aim is to have no aim. This can sound confusing and counterproductive to many in recent times with our need for physical truth and instant gratification we cannot reason with this understanding.

Many will have attempted to meditate after hearing of the amazing qualities it has to offer, but will quickly lose focus as not much seems to be happen when initiating the practice. We are told to focus on the breath as this is something we can perform both consciously and subconsciously – for when we are not focused on our breathing its carries on regardless, just like our digestive system takes the sustenance we ingest and turns it into energy or our heart pumps the life source around our bodies and we trust it to do so. But when it comes to our breathing we can have a say in this at any time we so wish. We can take a deep breath in with intent and this is why we are taught to do so when commencing meditation as it links the two parts of our mind, allowing for a bring together of the minds.

It also opens the gateway for our spiritual self to enter, no person can meditate without thinking thoughts, this is another hang up we all have and gives the self-critical idea we must be doing it all wrong as a result. It is only our focus upon these thoughts that stifles the process. The easiest way to describe how to approach our thoughts at these moments is to picture each one as a passing cloud, allow yourself to observe it but try not get to be fixated on it, let it pass! just as the wind helps the passing of the clouds, making way for the next thought to come into focus.

It is only when we fix our minds on the thought, that we lose our focus, be at peace with it and with yourself, don't throw the baby out with the bath water so to speak. Don't be too hard on yourself and try too hard, like the desire paradox! if you are desiring too much and told not to desire, do not then proceed to desire not to desire? Simply choose the middle way.

Bringing the chakras back into focus, we can also choose to concentrate and direct our attention away from the breath slightly and onto each energy wheel carrying out a complete body scan starting with the feet, moving up in your mind to the legs, hips and base of the spine. Once there we can imagine the colour of the root chakra and picture the connection it is making with the ground, helping ourselves to lose the negative energy pent up inside our bodies. This can help us find stability and a sense of purpose and so on as we move up the body.

When we reach the third eye and crown chakras we can take our spirituality to a higher level. If at this point you don't feel it necessary to do so and are content with your lot, then maybe meditation is all that's required to gain balance in your life. On the other hand if you feel something is missing - whether that be truth or even direction - then opening the third eye may just reveal exactly what you have been searching for. This is not to be taken lightly and can have some significant side effects, certain truths you may not wish to have been shown. There can be physical side effects too, namely a feeling of pressure in the forehead and a slight throbbing of the temples! Many have speculated that our modern living has impaired our ability to open the third eye through the calcification of the pineal gland through the many substances we incorporate into our diets and the additives present in the food and water we consume, which might have also be the reason behind some of the sleep depravity we encounter throughout our lives.

You may or may not be aware of the theory behind opening the third eye chakra. You might have heard the positives or been fearful of the negatives. Once again just like meditation you should go into this practice with an openness but without a wish to gain from it, therefore go about it purposefully but without purpose!

Certain people treat the opening of the third eye with an association of opening Pandora's box. For once opened it cannot be fully closed! but it will not be evil emitting from it only truth. It only serves to peel back the veil from our mind's eye, there may be things revealed to you that you would rather not wish to know, this is the epitome of ignorance is bliss! For when we are given knowledge it is extremely difficult to forget such things, but once you have transcended on this journey you will have a sudden realisation as to the reasons why you started out on this specific trek. The most attainable way to achieve this is through practice and repetition.

Whilst meditating, your concentration should be on the third eye chakra and then with closed eyes slowly focus on the centre of the forehead, between the brows, a slight strain and tension will be felt as a result. At this point picture in your mind the crown chakra opening up like the petals of a flower allowing for a brilliant white light to enter and meet the indigo colours of the mind's eye. Also having a light source (a candle's flame for instance) to focus on will aid in assisting and enhancing the intensity of the experience, now allowing your attention to return to the breath, imagine that you are breathing in a swirling cloud of deep blues and violets. This will form a connection thus bringing about the opening of the third eye, stay with this for as long as you need, then you can simply reverse the process or if you feel it necessary you can always imagine leaving the third eye slightly ajar - this is of course a personal preference.

Over time you will come to the conclusion that the beliefs you held dear may not be as clear-cut as first perceived. The whole world and indeed universe will open up to you as you have opened up to it – you will feel as though you are the only sober member of a drunken party in which everybody is talking but no one is really listening! You will be able to see things as they are and in their purest form, without preconceptions or prejudices. You will be transformed into an empowered empath who embraces the good and shuns the bad.

Initially it is a lot to conceptualise, a sadness mixed with anger can be the first emotions to surface as you become more aware of the injustices all around. A mental conflict of how things should be and the actuality of how things are can cause internal turmoil. We seek change, a change in the circumstances that surround us; of that we can control, but we also seek a change in the consciousness of those around us and feel an instinctive need for this! At this point you should remember that people need to arrive at this destination by their own volition, and to force such a thing onto them will only serve as a barrier, this feeling will subside so long as you trust in the process.

The next thing to take place is the witnessing of alignments at every junction in your life, this can come with relative frequency and the past coincidences can start to actually make sense, even the trials and tribulations are met with open arms and a wry smile and shrugged shoulders as you ask yourself 'what is the lesson now', like an eager student in their favourite class. Everything seems to come together as there appears to have been a method to the madness all along. You start to believe with every cell of your being that manifestations really do happen, next you will begin to question our own reality, so this begs the question can we really create that explicit experience we call reality? if we wish for something can it be said that if it is developed in our consciousness is it then more likely to occur as a result? This is our spiritual awakening!

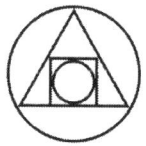

PART OF THE UNIVERSE

Your first introduction to the universe could very well have been Carl Sagen's brilliant documentary series 'Cosmos: A Personal Voyage', an awe inspiring truth of events, or you might have concocted your own ideas to the inner workings of this infinite realm. A seemingly impossible to grasp but also amazingly insightful scientific field which explores these very specific workings of the cosmos and that of our reality is quantum physics!

Quantum physics and its subsidiary, quantum mechanics, is arguably the most intriguing but conceptually difficult scientific field around. Many brilliantly minded scientists have contemplated quantum theory, some have excelled whilst many have failed to prove or explain this precarious field of topics, it may be a personal preference which has caused many to agree or disagree with certain findings. Scientists such as Schroedinger, Borh, Heisenberg and even Einstein spent many years researching and experimenting to find the truth behind this most incomputable of theories, so what is quantum physics and why is it so important? The simple answer is, it is the physics that explains how everything works, the way of explaining how the nature of particles that make up matter and the forces that interact with them, a fascinating window into the properties and mechanical workings of our universe.

The double slit experiment

Before delving into this most fascinating of experiments it is extremely important to firstly point out that the theory and workings behind this hypothesis can seem convoluted and a little difficult to conceptualize and that's okay, as the reason for its inclusion is to merely show that everything in our reality is the result of a conscious observation as opposed to a collection of probabilities, although there are a few academics who feel the experiment to be that of a contrived nature. The double slit experiment demonstrates the inseparability of the wave and particle natures of light and other quantum particles. The first to theorise and conduct this experiment was Thomas Young back in 1803, although some in the field will contest that Sir Isaac Newton had performed a similar experiment.

The test was to see if light photons act as a wave or that of a particle, (this being known as the Young experiment) and if the very observation could have an impact thus changing the outcome or even behaviour of said photons. This has been a conundrum for theorists over the last few centuries. This experiment involved particle beams of coherent waves passing through two closely spaced slits, the purpose being to measure the resulting impact on an impression screen directly behind. This has been tweaked and advanced in more recent times, even altering the format to capture more intrinsic data, but the simple premise to this being, will the screen behind display two horizontal lines of particles as you would expect as no interference should occur and if you would get an interference pattern displayed by the photons which should in theory act as a wave or something else! Perhaps they would behave like that of a wavicle?

If a wave pattern was observed, the resulting data will conclude that interference had been apparent and so the photons behaving like a wave would be true and two horizontal lines would indicate particles behave as theorised without interference. Due to the nature of the experimental world many derivatives took place. Now with the use of micro laser cutting edge machinery and indeed ever more directionally definitive lasers themselves coupled with better and more accurate testing equipment, scientists have been able to play devil's advocate as to alter the state of each test minutely but profoundly in each case. They soon became aware that both the photons and particles behaved in exactly the same way. This puzzled the scientists greatly. The biggest revelation being that the particles interfered with each other thus acting as a wave. This test was first carried out in a sealed box under no observation. Then they did a similar test with both photons and particles with an observational instrument to try to witness the photons as you would expect to interfere with each other as they passed through each slit. The results? They started behaving like particles, resulting in the formation of two horizontal lines on the screen behind, not progressively darker towards the middle and lighter towards the outsides (diffraction). This caused immense confusion. The fact there was a conscious observational instrument seemed to collapse the wave function of the photons and so they started isolating each component of the test.

First firing a single photon and in a different test, a single particle one at a time through the double slit slid once under no observation and once under observation respectively, the results? Nothing changed. The screen either had two horizontal lines if observed for both or an interference pattern if the experiment had not been witnessed, an unfathomable collection of data no doubt. This also meant that each particle or photon had to have passed through each slit simultaneously to have interfered with itself if a wave pattern was still seen when it had not been consciously observed. They also placed the observing instruments before and after the slits to see if this had any impact. They were perplexed to realise that even if the camera was observing past the slits the particles and photons seemingly reverted to an observable state thus going back in time (not literally but given the data the only rational explanation for it). Many argue the full meaning behind the experiment! as no definitive answer has been concluded and everything in this quantum field at present is either all conjecture or subjective to the expert!

You might not have even been privy to such studies and if you have managed to get your head around the last literature you might now be asking what is the point of such insert! Although this has vast implications with regards to quantum studies it also could have tremendous meaning for all humanity. It could be classed as the most compelling evidence towards and favouring a collective conscious, and so a universal consciousness. As you are probably already aware an atom is mostly made up of space, a proton, a nucleus and with an electron circling the nucleus, but the rest (hypothetically 99.9999%) is space with the addition of electromagnetic fields, what you are, what a tree is or a seemingly solid steel box is little more than space with theorized electromagnetic force fields, yet just because it is felt and is tangible this still should not crossover this point! Our visible spectrum is small in comparison to the vast ranges, but what we conceive to be our tangible reality is fashioned by the mind via in the input and interactions of the senses. The realest part of reality is that 99.9999% (variable) of anything is not simply made up of matter only force fields and probabilities (although this space can be occupied) so, what you imagine and believe to be real is in a sense only real in your perceived mind after your conscious awareness. Think of a chain link fence, you could make that metal wire extremely slender and from a distance it would be difficult to observe yet if you were to attempt to walk through it you could not as long as it held its integrity.

An electron once believed to be at one place whizzing around an atom in an orbit cannot be predicted as to where exactly it is placed, it can only have a probability and so in theory could be simultaneously at many points around the nucleus at any one time it is only in the conscious observation that the wave function collapses and it is seen at a point. This means everything around you and in space is just a collection of probabilities, it is only in the observation that they are so. Albert Einstein could not allow himself to commit to this argument and spent many years trying to find an alternative answer, once stating, "I like to think the moon is there even if I am not looking". Although he did coin the phrase, "reality is merely an illusion albeit a very persistent one", meaning reality is just a perceived version of things, it has nothing to do with universal truth! So going back to the statement, he is saying and possibly poking fun at the theory by stating if I am not looking at the moon you are telling me at that point it is not so? And the reply could be how can you know for sure it is still there if you are not actually observing it through your own eyes (which can seem a bit of a get out of jail free card)? You could say, "well the person next to me is viewing it and is whispering to me that it is so"! Yes but that person is consciously observing and is therefore collapsing the wave function and so a direct part of the collective conscious!

The most mind puzzling aspect to this is that if it is a categoric truth that a big bang took place, as to what was observing these series of events in order for it to be so? Was it the Tao? Was it the universe itself? Was it all of these and more? Just as you are made up of space dust your spiritual energy must originate and belong to all that is! It is hard for a person to conceive the difference between the mind, body and spirit. The body although made up of oxygen, carbon, hydrogen, nitrogen and calcium to the tune of 99% and the other 1% made up of other elements such as potassium, sulphur, sodium, chloride and magnesium, yet because it is fluid and soft we take ourselves and the flora, fauna outside the realm of being made up of just simply rocks and dust, we spill our life force when injured. How can we be biologically similar to a space rock? We function, we have a mind, we are different! This is the "I" talking! yes we are all blessed with intelligence, a mind, a will but deep down at the basic level physically you are the universe. You are made up in this life from base elements with a couple of buckets of water mixed in for good measure, this is the incredible thing, the fact you are the essence of this universe, you are the person you see on your way to work every morning, you are your noisy neighbour or the person you quarrel with sometimes at work, think of yourself as a cell in the universal body therefore surely working towards a common cause is the reason we are here, not to hinder or stifle others on their path! Arguments, fallouts, conflicts, assisting in greed, in corruption! Call it the devil on your shoulder, call it the snake in the Garden of Eden, call it what you like but know it is the ego that is the cause of all of that is wrong with humanity.

Life does not need to be heaven on earth or a godly paradise like an oasis in the barren desert! It has to help you grow and so naturally occurring hardships are of the utmost importance whether we like that fact or not. But then why if that is our goal to live a heavenly existence would humanity feel the overwhelming desire to control, divide and conquer, why make it harder than it has to be, does this not feel hypocritical? Positives and negatives, rights and wrongs, good and bad, love and hate, light and dark, a balance is always met but that doesn't have to be 50/50 for the most favourable of the two should always weigh the most! We can't help but feel that in recent times the balance is hanging precariously towards the dark side and so an awakening which does seem to have some pockets opening up around the world must and will come to fruition, not with a need but with a will to bring about change. A deeper understanding and connection should and will indeed be found once the smokescreen has been lifted and we see ourselves in others as we do the reflection in our mind's mirror. Whatever your stance, we all gravitate towards the innocent, the underdog, the honest and humble the genuine beings because a beautiful soul matters more to us deep down than anything else! Materialism and aesthetics distort this view. Try to observe the universe and all that is around you from a non-judgemental standpoint, to watch but not cast aspersions, have empathy and understanding for all that exists. We see the innocence of infants or animals and this warms our soul. We feel instant empathy towards them and sympathy when they are abused. Now let's flip this!

Say a cat scratches you, your first reaction is you think it had a will and is probably just a nasty cat. True, cats can show a range of emotions and are intelligent creatures, but all that cat is displaying is an instinctive defence response via a feedback loop. However, because it is felt on a personal level we cast aspersions onto that animal. We can think of them as selfish because (although not true of the behaviour of all cats if they have been interacted with humanely!) they do seem to only show a greater amount of affection towards their guardian when they require something, namely food, and comfort. Once again these are instincts. In the same way a baby crying teaches them that gaining attention through less than favourable behaviours brings about love and sustenance, the so-called play fighting with our pets isn't an exact science and even though seen with light humour, a fun activity for ourselves and the pet who appears to display the same actions towards their rival siblings can be pushed to the limit and cause a poignant reaction later down the line in the animal with which trust issues can develop, so might become wary of this and may interpret certain actions in a negative light. Very much like humans, it is instinctual and learnt behaviour with the small exception that we are fully aware of who we are and the possible repercussions of our actions. Maybe it is time we looked at all humanity in the same light. We see animals for the most parts with no predispositions or prejudices, with hope instead of disdain. We are too quick to find fault or put up barriers with people and the true nature of our connections become impeded, therefore we shouldn't try to write the story without first opening to a blank page. Nothing in this world is inherently good or bad, only our conceptualisation of things! this is true, but in the same breath only conscious determination can make it so.

Reverting back to Buddhism, Buddhists believe our spirit may take on many forms and live many lives (reincarnation) but only escape this cycle when nirvana has been achieved, only then can our spirit turn to light and return to the universe (enlightenment and ascension) you can either believe this or not. The theory behind reincarnation is as follows, you were born out of this world to live a life, show growth or not, and once you pass over you are reborn into a new life with a karmic aspect. Maybe you lived a wholesome life the first time, but still need to acquire vast amounts of knowledge or hardship for that spiritual growth to continue. On the other side you might have lived a life of luxury which caused greed, corruption and more of a materialistic aspect to your higher self. This might be seen as though you have missed the message entirely and on and on till the reason becomes apparent and the message is fully understood in which the truth prevails and steps towards enlightenment are within sight.

The striking aspects are how can you continue to edge closer if you are not aware of the previous life? This would be a reasonable question to ask and one that is backed up with another theory – that being upon death a significant amount of DMT is released which may serve to wipe or distort the memory and assist in the possibly deemed harrowing or confusing passing. DMT (N, N-Dimethyltryptamine) being a substance the human body produces naturally, but is also found in many natural sources, from certain psilocybin mushrooms to ayahuasca it has even been attempted to be synthesised.

The hallucinogenic properties of DMT are supposed to have profound effects on the human consciousness although a certain consensus shows that it might be harmful. Certain groups believe it is released when we dream to help us make sense of our life, while some believe it is behind all the near-death experiences encountered by people. Whatever the case there is no doubt that it is used to effect people at certain times in their life. It is illegal to consume DMT from organic sources in most countries yet has been proven to be present in the human body! Trace amounts have been discovered in the pineal gland and even neurons. Undeniably it is naturally produced by humanity as a species so this theory of the DMT assisting but also wiping our previous experiences seems pretty counterproductive, you may say that's because the meaning has to be found organically without a motive or a prior objective.

There are many ways to rediscover that knowledge, it is only our connection that has to be strengthened for glimmers to be shown. That is why meditation, beauty in others and one that we already bear witness to on a regular basis - nature! Is so important.

The world around us is the loudest whisper and biggest spiritually uplifting exercise we have at our disposal. It could be a walk in the park or often navigated quaint little quiet path, dispersing the golden sands between your toes on a sun kissed beach, hearing the waves lap across the shore line, watching the glistening silhouettes of sunlight dance on the water surface, climbing a hilltop to gain a vantage point in which to witness the unfolding rolling landscape of unimaginable beauty, to gazing up at the night sky enveloped by the warm wind drifting across your face with wonderments in your eyes and the myriad of sounds the nightlife plays like natures very own orchestra performing just for you. Isn't this life? To be exactly in the moment, cherishing every minute aspect and savouring the present, this is total connection!

When pondering life's meaning take this as your answer, to observe the universe in all its splendour, see it! Smell it! Hear it! Search it! But also truly feel it with every fibre of your body it should never be a question of why? but more a question of how! With the same compassion and intrigue an inspired five year old shows when also immersed in nature! it is only when you understand this that balance will swing away from the bad and life will once again become a blessing not a feat of endurance. What becomes more apparent at this time is that your awareness of the resonance inside you will increase. You will sense that your own vibration has been heightened and a calming symbiosis of the mind body spirit will be felt. Nikola Tesla famously said, "if you wish to understand the universe think of energy, frequency and vibration". This is a monumentally important statement! The meaning is quite simple, he was trying to tell us that everything in our universe has energy and as a result of that everything surely must have a vibration and frequency unique to that energy, a resonance! The enormity of what he told us opened up a whole new understanding of the cosmos. So what implications can this have on humanity? Everything made up of matter also has energy and must also vibrate with the emittance of a frequency due to the oscillation of atoms, and so we humans must therefore emit an overall frequency -the Schumann resonance. Winifreid Otto Schumann was a German physicist who predicted the resonance of the earth (its pulse). Whilst giving a lecture to his students he asked them to make a calculation of what the frequency between the earth and the Ionosphere was, without himself having the resulting data he would also attempt this equation and came to the conclusion that the frequency, although fluctuations occur, was precisely 7.83 hertz. This was forgotten until a few years later when approached to continue his study. He made a startling discovery! It was found that the resonance (once again with fluctuations) of the human body was also the very same frequency 7.83 hertz of the earth. So what does all this mean? It may give a new understanding to how our atmosphere and environments interact with our own low frequency electromagnetic energy. The SR is the result of solar radiation and lightning storms around the globe at any one time (a ball within a ball) and the electrical interference between. As the earth rotates and the day turns to night at a given coordinate the Ionosphere thins out and the frequency alters slightly. Could this then give rise to another element in regards to the human circadian rhythm as opposed to relying solely on the light/dark spectrum being interpreted and perceived by the eyes then signalled to the pineal gland? When human brain trials have been conducted via an EEG machine it has shown that different brainwaves quite obviously produce different frequencies. Our brainwaves are as follows: Delta 0.5-4 Hz, Theta 4-8 Hz, Alpha 8-13Hz, Beta 13-32Hz, Gamma 32-100Hz, each having a powerful role in how we think, process, relax, create and rejuvenate, they cause altered states of consciousness and can be regional in the brain - the lower the frequency the less aware we are and the higher the frequency the more awareness we appear to have.

Delta waves enable us to enter a deep dreamless state, loss of bodily awareness and help to repair and rejuvenate.

Theta waves enable us to reduce our consciousness, enter dream state, deep meditation, insight and creativity.

Alpha waves are emitted when we are physically and mentally relaxed.

Beta waves are produced when we are fully awake, alert, conscious thinking and excited.

Gamma waves are produced when we have a heightened perception, we are learning, problem-solving tasks, cognitive processing.

Whether coincidental or not - and we know what we think about coincidences - the Schumann resonance would therefore create brain entrainment at the precipice of the Theta waves and upon entering

Alpha waves. So this frequency has given rise to the belief that it increases cerebral blood flow, helps a person enter a higher level of hypnotisability and meditative state! For millennia, the OM Chant has been used to enhance our meditative mind state and just so happens to emit the very same inaudible frequency as SR. The theory of SR and its influence on people as a species is that this pulse helps enhance our psychological and physical wellbeing, and also helps us achieve our optimal brainwaves state. Humans and life itself may rely significantly on the frequencies below the earth's crust and the Ionosphere above to bring about an equilibrium, a Ying and Yang, although this harmony may just be getting disrupted slightly in this era we find ourselves due to the increase of ever expanding technology, which in turn might be causing an electromagnetic disturbance to exist, an observable increase in the pace of life and a decrease in overall wellbeing and harmony brought on by elevated anxiety and stress levels might be prevalent in these times.

So is there anything we can do to block this background noise and achieve a more serene existence in these heady times? Some holistic practices profess to a deeper knowledge. You will have heard of the healing qualities of quartz and the like, this crystal is said to heal the mind and body by emitting its own energy which can be absorbed by our perfect organism but this is only a pseudoscience as there is no factual evidence.

Quartz has very unique properties in the fact that it can turn vibrations into mechanical energy and vice versa. It also has a very stable resonance so that if you pass an electrical charge through the crystal it will vibrate at an accurate frequency consistently, hence its use in watchmaking for centuries to keep a steady pulse to emulate time. It therefore cannot simply heal a person through emitting energy, but it can serve as a placebo effect which is undoubtedly a positive for the human psyche. The only truth about the use of quartz is that it may be able to amplify and intensify our brainwaves in certain states if we are trying to achieve a meditative state of Theta brainwaves through a syncing of the frequencies and an echoing effect. This could have a magnifying beneficial outcome.

Another new age trend we see is the use of binaural beats to help you achieve these desired states, the principle being that whilst listening with the aid of headphones, tones are emitted with slightly differing frequencies from the left and right audio outlets for example 440 hertz to 446 hertz. The reasoning being that the two frequencies will have a cancelling effect interpreted by the brain and the remaining frequency of 6 hertz will result in brain entrainment forming (a syncing of our brainwaves to external frequencies). You may ask why not simply emit a monoaural beat? Or other types of constant inaudible tonal sounds to gain this desired effect? You possibly can and although the jury is out there maybe some truth to this practice. If evidence proves the effectiveness of binaural beats in time albeit many researchers show scepticism towards this new trend, the benefit it could have over monoaural beats is that it has the characteristic of audible relaxing tones which could work alongside the ultra-low frequency for an all-round greater outcome. As music is felt deeply and can change our emotional outlooks its properties are overwhelmingly positive.

Which brings us onto the emotional frequencies chart. We as a species resonate at between 5-10Hz (whole body) we have 5 brainwaves ranging from 0.5 Hz 100 Hz, (though typically 40Hz is our highest gamma range) our heart's electrical pulse is generated and the frequency from this amounts to 1Hz yet these spiritual charts show a range of between 0-1000 Hz with force embodying the bottom half ranges and power making up the top half. This could perhaps be true on a spiritual level but cannot possibly be true at an elementary level.

We cannot disprove the spiritual emotional significance as in time this may be shown to hold some water, as a truth today could just as easily be a false tomorrow and vice versa. If history has taught us anything it is that this sentence is one of the utmost importance, the problem arises in the fact that our brainwaves are electrically charged impulses and physically/emotionally we cannot produce these specific higher frequencies.

If this were true and we achieved our higher emotional states as dictated by the chart, in harmony with our highest possible brainwave state of gamma, this would tell us that we are in constant turmoil as the highest emotional state we could obtain would be that of fear and as we fell back to the lower frequency brainwaves, these emotions would turn to grief, apathy, guilt and shame - not a very happy existence at all. But it is worth reminding that if this goes towards helping people who believe this to be true and that we can indeed raise our vibrations, then this can be seen as a wonderful belief system nevertheless and will cause an advancement in the body and mind just by that sheer thought! We can however raise our vibration on a spiritual level by simply 'lifting our spirits'. The human body is a phenomenally complex organism. Our emotions are held and governed by the subconscious mind and this initiates various chemical releases from its interpretation of external influences and in this very process enables better connections to form throughout our neuropathic system and so helps a person gain the best experience from life and feel a stronger connection to the present. Everything is relative and everything in regards to emotions is either instinctive (learnt behaviour due to our circumstances) or our perceived interaction with the outside world. You can simply smile, even under mundane circumstances and this will cause a series of bodily chain reactions. It is in our awareness and conscious reactions that we can change to a more symbiotic relationship with life.

There are no real emotions just 'it' 'the universe' 'the Tao' emotions assist you by helping you to feel this reality deeply and gain the most from it, They are chemical messages that convey sometimes subtle, and sometimes powerfully felt/perceived sensations, yet spiritually we have the undeniable sense of good and bad, a spectrum of morality. If only there was a transparent spectrum to see the beauty within, how different would our lives be? And so if there are no real coincidences, just a conscious course, then surely having moral intentions will only serve you, and immoral intentions will only serve to inflict suffering and pain.

Everything in this universe must have some basic level of consciousness. Yes your belief system at this very moment is telling you to question inanimate objects such as a rock or a steel chair leg, yet even those base minerals and elements on a sub atomic scale has to have a conscious process, if not then why are they constructed in such a unified way? What causes the electron to circumnavigate the nucleus? A valid answer could be simply the laws of the universe! to which the reply would be, exactly!

People need hard factual evidence before they can accept something with ease and have a tendency to dispel all other theories unless hope is a part of the process. On this planet it would be a fair assessment to say that life can only come from life, true, right? But this cannot always have been so! we are given the theory of the big bang and base elemental reactions. In the same fashion we only truly believe that life is the only source of pure consciousness and think of the start of the universe as just a strange happening without the consideration that there had to have been a will, therefore conscious determination which is a paradox in itself, a rudimental chicken and egg conundrum. The main psychological hang up is that we as beings try our hardest to fit all our beliefs into a tiny neat box with a pretty bow on it and then proceed to hold onto these fixed ideas with a persistent fear and threat of them being questioned. Sometimes, as honourable as it sounds, we are even willing to turn in our mortality card in exchange for keeping hold of this box, surely a broadening of the mind would lead to an acceptance and vaster amounts of feasibility regarding certain topics? True knowledge is in the knowing you ultimately know nothing! Does this not sound evermore profound? You might start to understand this as less cryptic and an actuality now.

To tightly grip one set of creeds and shun all others will always have a narrowing, tapering off effect on the mind, and so an openness to all is a much more favourable adventure to take and a powerful seeker of truth. Many theories will turn up wrong but all it takes is for one to have been right for the journey to have been a success. We dream up things that seem impossible and yet in time we come to realise this not to be true, all things in time are possible, it is our closed off fixed beliefs that push this further from reality.

We have been given an amazing gift of higher consciousness and yet many through no fault of their own choose to live a life governed entirely by instinct and emotions with their lower self in the driving seat, try to get to know yourself first! if you are anything you are the universe reflecting upon itself through the cosmic mirror and what the universe does not know might not be worth knowing.

You might have found certain aspects to be that of a repetitive nature, they have not been erroneously left throughout the thread or misplaced. They are there to form and serve as the backdrop to the narrative thus emphasize the underlying message to the story of our misgivings and plights of life therefore aiding in the breaking of the chains, so that you yourself might be able to inflict an internal liberation.

JUST BE!

You are enough! Everything you wish to be resides within you, there is no need to search for excellence so, peel back this fabricated outer shell to reveal the perfection that already exists. Of course you can study harder and accrue vast knowledge, you can body build to achieve greater levels of strength or train to run marathons to increase endurance and push the limits, but your paradigm of obtaining immaculate magnificence will always appear further away like a mirage in the desert. Be mindful of your drive, think less and know more!

You have to appreciate the already near perfection and oneness you are, so enjoy this most fortunate of events, not with a fear of not becoming the best or achieving greatness, but with a quiet sensibility. We as a species have to learn to inhale/exhale again fully! as this most natural of processes has become impaired of late we are forever trying to hold onto our breath as we do with life and in exactly the same way we find ourselves in danger and hesitant to make a sound, It's almost as if we are waiting for life to find and embrace us! but with a suffocating dread hence, we stay hidden in our very own metaphoric nook, conscious that at any moment the impending doom of unfortunate circumstances will seek us out. A constant battle fought with anxiety, failure and rejection, a missing sense of accomplishment, let that breath out! You are totally fine! just as you are, never should you feel insignificant or powerless!

In fact you are better than fine, you are you, a unique slither of the universe. There is no one quite like you! It is that quirkiness which radiates beauty, it will never be the mundaneness of conformity so relax and ask yourself, "what pressure?".

By trying to hold onto the reins of life and navigate it as a jockey tries to navigate the race course and steer the horse in its every movement, in that very action we forget to fully experience the magic as we are so preoccupied with just trying to stay in the saddle and hold on for dear life with every hurdle we have to scale. Also do not spend your life searching for the pot of gold to discover, it was inside you all along! live presently with your thoughts and ask yourself this question, "will this serve me and my immediate needs?"

Once you have your answer only then press ahead with conviction! If it feels right, you should entitle yourself to carry the task out irrespective of burden. Use all that is around you, dance with life, become intertwined with it, be the Capoeira dancer and take life as your partner, learn to flow. It is only human interference that alters the universal path. If only we sat back and allowed events to unfold unrestricted, would we then see that all the fighting and controlling was the very thing that hindered our road to success. Sometimes, the harder we try the harder the thing becomes to perform and distorts the process. When we forget a thought in our minds the more we struggle with retrieving said thought and the more it is lost! It is only when we forget to try that the secret is finally revealed, sometimes it is a simple explanation as we just can't see the wood for the trees! The hardest concept to try to understand is 'don't try! But don't try not to try!' just do.

You should also be aware of external influences having an effect on your understandings - they may alter your perception of what life is all about, striving, going beyond, going beyond what exactly? The last person to achieve something great? Outdoing each other? Letting self-righteousness get in the way as you look within and ask what is my life? What is life? Ruminate and give your spirit time to answer this question, you will fully appreciate what the answer ought to be! Life is life, life is to be lived, not held but nurtured and most of all experienced in its entirety, become engrossed in the now! Do tasks purposefully whether it be simple things such as taking a shower, ironing clothes, washing the dishes, or intimate meaningful actions such as playing with your children, enjoying a party or a meal, taking part in your favourite craft or hobby, become fully immersed in the activity.

Allow thoughts to flow! When the mind is of a stillness akin to the water in a mill pond only then will you see them as a series of clouds falling over you in a slow ebbing manner and begin to see clearly again and efficiently work through each with serenity. The subconscious mind is a brilliant worker but a lousy task master, so use its strengths but try not to let it use you!

For the most part, animals (depending on their intelligence) rarely think, they are driven primarily by instincts. Although the higher up the cognitive ladder you climb, i.e. certain mammals such as dolphins and great apes who fall into our category to some extent, yet take a crocodile for instance rarely do they contemplate an action they just do! embodying the act, a vast amount of their governing body is dictated by the instinct to survive. We too can allow ourselves to become one with our environment and enter this flow state, and in turn gain the key to the autonomy of our minds and body to perform specific tasks. Taoism – Wu Wei – non action – flowy – natural course, the way!

Often disputed to have been somewhat of a legend, the founder of this philosophical movement was Lao Tzu (meaning master). He is said to have resided in the village of Quran, in the district of Hu, in the state of Chu (the modern day eastern province of Henan). Although this myth has been contended for centuries, Lao Tzu is said to have lived in the 5th-6th BCE. An ancient Chinese philosopher and writer, his most notable book being *Tao Te Ching*, the original guide book to Taoism. It includes short verses regarding a number of central aspects of Taoism such as action-nonaction, the duality of nature, knowledge and virtue. It emphasises doing what is natural allowing the process to happen without force, going with the flow in accordance with the Tao. A universal force which flows through all things and connects and frees them, each verse and message is profound in nature and can help to teach all a simpler way of life. We can extrapolate four teachings from the Tao Te Ching to incorporate into our lives and so enter this very flow state.

- Simplicity, Patience, Compassion.
- Going with the flow – "When nothing is done nothing is undone."
- Letting go – "If you realize that all things change, there is nothing for you try to hold on to."
- Harmony.

If you become mindful of each of these doctrines then the results of integrating them within your daily rituals will be significant, some of the many quotes to always have in the back of your mind are as follows.

- "When you let go of what you are, you may become what you might be."
- "If you do not change direction you may end up where you are heading."
- "Kindness in words creates confidence, kindness in thinking creates profoundness and kindness in giving creates love."
- "Love is of all our passions the strongest, for it attacks simultaneously the head the heart and the senses."
- "Silence is a source of great strength."
- "From caring comes courage."

And lastly, "when you are content to be simply yourself and don't compare or compete, everybody will respect you".

It is hard for the western world to fully accept these ancient eastern proverbs because the literary translation for the Chinese language shows greater emotions and thoughts and cannot simply be translated in its complexity to other western cultures, hence a lot of poignancy can be lost in the act.

Higher self / Lower Self

Higher self = Spirit = Positivity provides nourishment.

Lower self = Ego = Negativity provides nourishment.

We think of self-confidence as deriving from the ego. Although the truth is, self-confidence comes from connecting with who we really are and appreciating our worth and unique qualities.

The ego makes you question yourself. It is your own personal critic causing you to feel less, comparing you to others. It can be seen as a protective armour we wear in times of peace, only serving to weigh us down. It may be wiser for you to leave your ego at the door and enter into life completely. Always remember what is important and what is not, our hang ups about the future are often unwarranted so why go through the unprecedented pain twice?.

Humanity has two very distinctive and peculiar emotional states also born out of this false self, that of shame and of guilt, two mystifying human emotional traits. We should never feel guilty or shame only admiration for enduring the pain. When we take ourselves too seriously we can prolong the agony so be spontaneous, perform random acts of love and humour as this will help alleviate the depressive moments. We have to learn to start loving each other again and show unrelenting compassion. Be the first to offer an olive branch, also try not to get too attached to your reality just allow it to wash over you and give yourself the chance to receive it fully. A minimalistic approach to life could assist with this attachment you feel at times! Fall back and let the Tao guide you, for once you were blind and now you see.

Gratitude and affirmations

The theory of affirmations can feel farfetched to the unwitting eye, but the simple truth is affirmations do work! The factual reasoning affirmations work is all down to positively re-enforced repetition. Just as our subconscious mind can domineer us emotionally, we can choose to dictate those emotions by applying positive feedback, and over time a new neurological pathway can be formed, in return a stronger connection will be made. A simple way to show this is by forming a smile with your mouth and lips, even when we are not elated! Our brains will interpret this and release a higher quantity of serotonin and thus a chain reaction will occur. A happy state will breed a happier state and so this is something to remember the next time you are feeling down, because of this very fact when we are having a hard time of it, we can fall into the trap of moaning and spreading negative thoughts, this is the main culprit to making our bad days worse, it is all down to our mental input/output exchange. So, showing gratitude for all you are and all you have, who knows, you might just get much more than you bargained for!

When you think the thoughts and wishes with a positive mindset and stay within that proximity what will be will be also, the opposite is true! Remember they who think they can and they who think they cannot, are both right! The universe will endeavour to make that happen, a what, why or where should not matter. In the same breath you should not wish to want in this life! Nor should you wish to want to lose anything you already possess – no desire.

Get back to the wonderment and appreciation you had when you were a child, over the years this will have waned, but this doesn't have to be so. There is one more thing we all seem to do and that is hold onto regret which can be said to be a pointless exercise, whether we become regretful of mistakes we have made, lost opportunities through chances we should have taken! You as a person can and do have a big influence on your life and the environment around you but that conceived influence you think is far less than you can imagine.

Here is a brilliant story to emphasise that fact and it will go some way to help you to visualise this conveyed message that things happen for a reason and should be viewed in that way, for only time will display the reason why it came to be so. An ancient fable as retold by the brilliant Alan Watts.

The Chinese Farmer

Once upon a time there was a Chinese farmer who lost a horse that had ran away. All his neighbours came round that evening and said to him, "That's too bad" to which he replied, "Maybe". The next day the horse came back and brought several wild horses with it. And all the neighbours gathered around that night and said, "Well that's great isn't it?" and he said, "Maybe". The very next day his son was attempting to tame one of the wild horses, was riding it and was thrown from the horse and broke his leg and all the neighbours came round that evening and said, "Well that's too bad isn't it?" and the farmer said, "Maybe".

The next day the conscription officers came round looking for people for the army and rejected his son because of his broken leg. And again all the farmer's neighbours came around that night and said, "Isn't that wonderful?" and he replied, "Maybe".

The whole process of nature is an integrated process of immense complexity and it is really impossible to tell whether anything that happens in it is good or bad. Because you never know what will be the consequences of a misfortune or you never know the consequences of good fortune. Be careful what you wish for, isn't that what we are told? Time is a great healer when mistakes are made by you or others an extremely simple process should be adhered to!

Picture a time you have dropped a soda bottle on the floor what is the first thing you do? You sit it down somewhere to settle and after some time you proceed to open it slowly. This is the very act you should emulate when things have turned awry for you. Give it space and time, and then slowly proceed forward for this is the purest way of pressing ahead and not exacerbate your problems. Things happen for a reason, do not try to gain the answer instantly allow it to show itself when the time is right.

So, explore the possibilities, explore new horizons! But most importantly … learn to explore yourself!

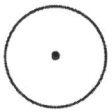

Printed in Great Britain
by Amazon